The Ericksonian Hypnosis Series. Volume 1: Phobias

Stephen Brooks

AND THE ART OF COMPASSIONATE ERICKSONIAN HYPNOTHERAPY

Volume 1: Phobias

Jos van Boxtel

Mindspring Publishing

Mindspring Publishing, Goeman Borgesiuslaan 77, 3515 ET Utrecht, The Netherlands. Mindspring.nl

Names: Jos van Boxtel – 1961 author.

Title: Stephen Brooks and the Art of Compassionate Ericksonian Hypnotherapy

Description: Mindspring Publishing 2020. Series: The Ericksonian Hypnosis Series; Volume 1: Phobias. Includes bibliographical references and index.

ISBN: 978-9-0830746-0-3 Stephen Brooks and the Art of Ericksonian Hypnotherapy (PAPERBACK PRINT).

Subjects: Mental health - Hypnotherapy – Hypnosis - Psychotherapy – Counselling - Clinical Psychology.

Photo credits: Gerard Helt: Jos van Boxtel. Chao Chirumpatareefah Na Champassakdi: Stephen Brooks.

Cover and interior design: Mindspring Publishing

Cover text set in Libre Baskerville, interior in Garamond 12.

Mindspring Publishing books are produced with environmental mindfulness.

Dedicated to Stephen Brooks' many students over the years.

For information about training with Stephen Brooks, please visit:

stephenbrookshypnosis.com

For information about training with Jos van Boxtel, please visit:

mindspringtraining.nl

Table of Contents

Introduction

I first became aware of Stephen Brooks in 2011, when I saw a video of a therapy demonstration recorded by the University of East Sussex in England in 1990. As a hypnotherapist, I had studied the work of Milton Erickson for several years but had never seen such an elegant and effective demonstration as the one given by Brooks in this video. I was struck by the ease and effectiveness with which he guided his client into different states of conscious awareness and through major therapeutic changes. I had to find out more about this Stephen Brooks, so I went on the Internet to check if he was still around. To my surprise, I discovered that he was offering training courses in the UK and I immediately signed up for one. Now, seven years later, I have studied his work intensively, become acquainted with him personally and currently cooperate with him in writing and teaching.

Stephen Brooks started his work in the mid-seventies when he became interested in hypnosis and began to study the work of Milton Erickson. During that time, Erickson had many followers in the United States, but in the UK, Brooks was the first to take notice of his work. Having access to only a handful of Erickson's research papers, Brooks had to rely on his own interpretation of Erickson's work to help him develop his personal style. He learned quickly and soon started helping people with personal problems of all kinds. He became increasingly successful; after only a few years, he was running a full-time practice treating patients from all over the UK. Much like Milton Erickson in his day, Brooks became the therapist to seek out when no one else could help. In 1979 Brooks founded British Hypnosis Research, the practice and training institute from which he treated thousands of clients and trained hundreds of students in the art of indirect hypnosis. When NLP came to the UK in the late seventies, he took training in it and incorporated it into his work. In 1995, he founded the British Society of Clinical and Medical Ericksonian Hypnosis.

Although extremely successful, Brooks wasn't satisfied with his work and life. Having been a practising Buddhist since the age of 14, he decided to move to Thailand to study Buddhist psychology. He wanted to find a way of integrating Buddhist principles with hypnosis and psychotherapy. After several years of study, introspection and meditation, he had enriched his work by creating an approach based on the principle of non-attachment.

In the course of his career, Brooks has given many, recorded, demonstrations for training purposes. On his courses he has always insisted on demonstrating therapy with clients he has never met before, in order to show how even a one-session treatment can help someone overcome severe problems such as phobias, obsessions, eating disorders or depression. Although Brooks' work has evolved over the last three decades, the recordings from the 1990s are fascinating. For the student of hypnosis, they are perhaps most useful as an introduction to his work as his skills and techniques have become increasingly subtle and implicit over the years, meaning that, although more helpful and powerful for the client, it is harder for the observer to analyse them. The earlier demonstrations are a little easier to break down and are therefore a good place to start studying his work. Still, it took me days of repeated and detailed study to understand and analyse the complexity of Brooks' communication with the client who is the subject of this book. A seemingly casual or humorous conversation turns out to be a complex, indirect and multilevel interaction, tailored to the client's problem, and thinking style and oriented towards their eventual goal. His contact with a client seems easy and relaxed, almost like a friendly chat. Nevertheless, his words are emphatic, compelling and challenging. His language is condensed, and every sentence contains multiple messages for the client; some are directed towards the conscious mind while others reach towards the unconscious mind. He carefully observes postures, movements and minimal expressions, always looking for messages from the unconscious mind. His own nonverbal communication is gentle yet powerful, playful yet serious. Every posture, gesture and movement he makes during a therapy session has a meaning and is there to help the client enter trance or take the next therapeutic step. Every change in voice tone, inflection, hesitation or pause is used for maximum effect. Brooks' early background as a musician and performer can be clearly recognised in his work as a therapist. His intense rapport and highly refined technique often enable him to resolve a problem in just a single session. In fact, he sets in motion an unconscious process that continues long after the session has finished. It is as if seeds are sown that lie dormant in the client's mind, only to blossom at the most appropriate and helpful time.

Brooks' success is not solely a result of his technique and talent. I think it has much to do with his attitude and lifestyle. He believes deeply that his clients have unconscious resources, natural healing capacity and a willingness to become better. He is always prepared to create a new technique —or adapt an existing one— and tailor it exactly to the client's needs. As he often says, "I fly by the seat of my pants. I never know what I am going to do for a client until I've almost done it. I work with what the client gives me moment by moment, albeit from a certain set of principles, techniques and language patterns."

Clearly, for Brooks, therapy is not just about helping someone overcome a symptom or problem; it is an opportunity to help each client have a healthy and rewarding life in a deeply compassionate way. Brooks thinks more with his heart than his head. His approach has evolved over many years but blossomed after his time in the jungles of northern Thailand.

Watching the recordings, I soon realised that a single minute of a session would provide enough material for an entire lecture and a full session would be enough to fill a book. This is how the idea of a series of books based on different problems came about.

This series provides a unique way to learn Stephen Brooks' innovative approach to therapy and how to apply it to various problems. Each book details his work with a single client with a specific symptom, problem, goal, frame of reference and personality. The analysed transcripts show how Brooks tunes into the client's issues, needs and beliefs, utilising all this information to induce trance and to create a therapeutic intervention. The transcripts also demonstrate how information gathering, rapport building, trance induction and therapy happen simultaneously and support each other. Each book in this series offers the reader a chance to study Brooks' work from a different perspective and in a different application.

The books are divided into two parts. The first is an overview of the hypnotherapeutic principles and techniques that are used in a particular session. The second part is the transcript of that session with a detailed analysis of it. The transcript is divided into sections that correspond to a step or phase in the therapeutic process. After each section, you will find an interpretation of what happened, explaining Brooks' verbal and nonverbal communication in relation to that of the client's. This is followed by a list of the various language patterns and techniques used. The aim is to break down the magic that occurs when Brooks works with clients and to make the principles, techniques and language patterns behind it available for personal study by students, clinicians and therapists.

Acknowledgements

I would like to thank Jack Deverson and Daniëlle Molenaar for proofreading this book and a special thanks to my friend and colleague Trish Smith for her valuable corrections, suggestions and ideas during the process of writing this book, as well as her general support to the BHRTI.

PART ONE

Principles
Techniques
Language patterns

Chapter 1: Principles

Ericksonian hypnotherapy is based on a set of principles. These principles are basic concepts relating to people, life, the mind, problems, trance, solutions and therapy. The principles a therapist adopts strongly influence his perception, orientation and communication when working with a client. The traditional model in medicine is based on the principle of diagnosis and treatment. This means a doctor first investigates the nature of a disease and then prescribes the corresponding medication, operation or another form of treatment. Psychotherapy, as it developed in the late 19th century, was based on these same principles and many current forms of psychotherapy still operate in this way. Brooks, however, rejected the model of diagnosis-treatment in psychotherapy early in his career. Instead, he uses a model based on the principle of observation and utilisation as developed by Milton Erickson. Rather than diagnosing a client, he carefully observes the client's responses and then utilises them to create a solution. The principle of observation-utilisation is at the heart of Ericksonian hypnotherapy and distinguishes it from any other form of psychotherapy.

Observation

Like Milton Erickson, Brooks is a master of observation. He carefully observes his clients, looking for changes in facial expression, gestures, movements, changes in breathing, blinking or any other discernible expression of the body. Each time a client talks, Brooks listens for changes in voice tone, the use of half sentences, mistakes, slips of the tongue and the use of metaphor or humour to express something or cover something up. He watches to see if facial expression, posture or gesture match the words being spoken (congruity) or reveal something different (incongruity). He is also aware that the client might reveal valuable information in the form of nonverbal metaphors. Brooks rarely writes down the information a client gives him. Instead, he immediately utilises the client's words or keeps them in the back of his mind to use later in the session.

Acceptance

Having observed the client's behaviour, the next step is that of full acceptance. Every expression, action, thought, feeling or belief is totally accepted as long as it is within the boundaries of safety, for both therapist and client. For Brooks, acceptance is an attitude, a state of mind he is in constantly, when working with a client. However irrational, abnormal, unconventional or delusional a client appears, he will accept him or her with all his heart. If a client judges or rejects his or her own behaviour Brooks will accept both the behaviour and the rejection of it. This leads to a rapid and strong rapport, which is the basis for all the work that follows. The principle of acceptance is not only important for building rapport, but it is also a prerequisite or part of the next principle: utilisation.

Utilisation

Utilisation is the principle that distinguishes Ericksonian hypnotherapy from any other therapeutic method. Whatever the client does, feels, thinks, or believes is used (utilised) for trance induction or problem-solving. Utilising the positive aspects of the client's own experience —such as learning, happy memories or exceptions to the problem— has become an integral part of various approaches like NLP and Solution Focused Therapy (De Shazer & Dolan, 2007) (O'hanlon & Weiner-Davis, 1989). Utilising the negative aspects, however, is an important characteristic of Ericksonian hypnotherapy. Problematic behaviours are not directly corrected or changed; they are utilised to change themselves. Resistance by the client is considered to be a way of communicating, not a problem; it is utilised to induce a state of trance or create therapeutic change. A limiting belief is utilised by being reformulated in such a way it contradicts itself or enhances therapeutic change. Brooks utilises anything the client presents —from momentary words, gestures or feelings to long-term beliefs, patterns or symptoms— to induce trance, solve problems and create a positive future.

Cooperation

In many therapeutic approaches, the client's cooperation is considered a prerequisite for successful therapy. If the client does not cooperate (is resistant), this needs to be discussed and resolved before therapy can start. Ericksonian hypnotherapy is different in the sense that cooperation is practically inevitable because everything the client thinks, feels, says or does is welcomed, accepted and utilised. The client can be critical, sceptical, resistant or even hostile; no matter what kind of attitude the client exhibits, it can be utilised for trance induction and therapeutic intervention. In fact, the client's behaviour, whatever it is, is considered to be an unconscious attempt to communicate with the therapist. Although this attempt might not be very elegant or constructive, interpreting it as cooperation builds rapport and helps the client to develop a more constructive, collaborative style.

Responsiveness

A general objective of Ericksonian hypnotherapy is to get the client to respond. Interventions are not chosen according to diagnosis; they are developed along the way, based on the client's response to each individual step. Unconscious responses outside of the client's usual behavioural repertoire are particularly evoked and stimulated. Brooks works according to this principle from the moment of his first contact with a client. His verbal and nonverbal communication aims to elicit or even provoke responses, hypnotically or therapeutically. If the client doesn't respond, Brooks will subtly change his course until he or she does. Any response —whether positive or negative— is welcomed, encouraged and seen as cooperation. Responsiveness is considered much more important than understanding the problem. Conscious understanding of the problem and the way to solve it can be a by-product of change rather than a prerequisite for it (as it is in Cognitive Therapy). In the end, Ericksonian hypnotherapy is about getting the client to think and act in a way that resolves problems and clears symptoms, promoting happiness, well-being and self-actualisation.

Flexibility

Ericksonian hypnotherapists should be flexible in their work with clients. Flexibility concerns all aspects of the therapeutic encounter, from general approach, techniques, goals and session length to the overall number of sessions. Ericksonians are flexible in their communication style, be it verbal, nonverbal, direct, indirect, hypnotic or non-hypnotic. They switch skilfully between the four layers of hypnotherapy: information gathering, rapport building, trance induction and therapeutic intervention. Symptoms are interpreted in terms of personal meaning and possible utilisation rather than predefined indicators of a disorder. Brooks is extremely flexible, always adapting himself to the client's needs, beliefs, and minimal cues as well as his own associations, insights and intuition. He seamlessly changes course when something doesn't seem to be working or when new information necessitates a different approach. Brooks is not just being flexible to help the client resolve his problem, he is also demonstrating it and teaching the client to be flexible in the way he communicates and behaves. The reason that clients are in therapy in the first place is that they lack the required flexibility to be successful and happy. The more flexible they become through therapy, the better equipped they are for future challenges.

Resource-oriented

Ericksonian hypnotherapy is resource-oriented. Milton Erickson considered the unconscious mind to be a vast reservoir of resources that have been acquired over a lifetime. Many of these resources, like the memory of learning to read and write, are taken for granted. Other resources have been forgotten or are not considered useful by the client. A basic principle in Ericksonian hypnotherapy is that the client already has whatever it takes to solve the problem, in the form of positive memories, learning experiences, capacities, talents, dreams etc. The hypnotherapist's job is to create a verbal and nonverbal context to activate these unconscious resources. Part of that is freeing the unconscious mind from conscious limitations and conscious control.

Unconscious change

In Ericksonian hypnotherapy, the unconscious mind plays a central role in solving problems and in changing a person's life for the better. In many therapeutic models, awareness is considered a prerequisite for change. In Cognitive Behavioural Therapy, for example, the client is encouraged to become aware of irrational beliefs, change them consciously and then practise expressing them in feelings and behaviour. In Ericksonian hypnotherapy we, more or less, do the opposite. Change happens unconsciously and is experiential rather than cognitive. The conscious mind is deliberately distracted, confused or overloaded to prevent it from analysing the therapist's suggestions and controlling unconscious responses. The role of the unconscious is emphasised by praising all of its functions and acknowledging its expression. By distracting the conscious and stimulating the unconscious, the latter can express itself, mobilise resources and resolve problems. Unconsciously, the client knows that he or she has solved the problem and can generalise the change to new contexts or events.

This process of generalisation can be enhanced during the session with suitable post-hypnotic suggestions.

Strategic

Ericksonian hypnotherapy is strategic in the sense that the hypnotherapist has a goal for the client in mind and a strategy for how to get there. The therapist takes responsibility for trance to develop (if hypnosis is used), and for therapeutic steps to be taken. Based on the client's verbal and nonverbal behaviour, he chooses which trance phenomena to elicit and which hypnotherapeutic techniques to use. The therapist leads, utilising the material the client offers him. Working strategically means defining a goal that encompasses and goes beyond the client's initial goal. Clients regularly come into therapy for the removal of a symptom like a phobia, obsession or addiction. They define their goal from a 'problem' perspective, using the limited scope of their conscious mind. Often, they don't realise that symptom resolution may involve a change in behaviour, affect, thinking style and beliefs. Furthermore, a client might unconsciously long for much more than just getting rid of the symptom but not consider this to be possible. As Carol Lankton puts it:

> "I frequently find that clients underrate their resources and tend to take a 'minimalist' route on their journeys through life; that is, they pack only the barest essentials of choices." (Zeig & Gilligan, 1990) [1]

Goal setting in Ericksonian hypnotherapy goes well beyond the NLP 'well-formed outcome' model, where the client defines his goal consciously and checks its reality through conscious evaluation. An Ericksonian hypnotherapist continuously looks and listens for unconscious messages —in the form of nonverbal cues, slips of the tongue, or client metaphors— to develop an idea about the client's actual goal: the goal that resonates with his or her unconscious resources, needs, dreams and potential. Brooks never limits himself to mere symptom removal or short-term goal achievement. He sets up his sessions to create a snowball effect that continues to improve the client's life, long after therapy has finished.

[1] Some clients do the opposite in creating unrealistically high goals and thus set themselves up for failure.

Naturalistic

Ericksonian hypnotherapy is naturalistic in the sense that it draws upon natural, commonplace experiences. Trance is considered to be a normal state that is evoked easily in daily life. Brooks induces and utilises these states extensively in his work. In his demonstrations, he often builds on this natural trance-ability. Hypnotic phenomena —such as amnesia, dissociation, catalepsy and regression— are also seen as natural behaviours that occur in moments of intense focus, daydreaming, surprise, confusion or shock. For example, someone may freeze (i.e. become cataleptic) if startled. Going into a trance-like state, solving problems and reaching goals are all, natural capacities. Everyone has at some time overcome difficulties, solved problems and reached goals and so every client has the ability to do so. And even if someone does not believe they have such experiences, they can fantasise about it or identify with someone who has. Brooks utilises natural associations, mechanisms and potentials to help clients enter states of trance and solve their problems. The naturalistic approach distinguishes Ericksonian hypnotherapy sharply from traditional hypnotherapy, which uses standardised rituals for induction and symptom-based scripts for therapy.

Systemic

Ericksonian hypnotherapy is systemic in nature. Working systemically means including the client's social system, which can be their current family, their extended family or their family of origin. This is often necessary because people are social beings whose patterns, beliefs, needs, problems and goals are influenced if not governed by the system they are a part of. Any change in a client's social behaviour will affect the system, directly or indirectly and positively or negatively. Some family members might welcome and support problem resolution while others may resist it or try to reverse it. Both the client and their family members might benefit from maintaining a symptom or be afraid of what will happen when it is gone. Many systemic therapies, e.g. Brief Therapy, directly involve family members in the therapy process. In Family Reconstruction, as developed by Virginia Satir, family members are role played by participants of a therapy group (Nerin, 1986). Brooks was trained directly by Satir in the 1980's and integrated her approach with his Ericksonian roots. Rather than using the group technique, he worked hypnotically to elicit and reorganise the client's internalised family system. Later he enriched his hypnotic and systemic approach with the principle of non-attachment, allowing clients to resolve the basic spiritual cause of problems and empowering them to grow way beyond the ties of family, professional organisation or society.

Rapport

In Ericksonian hypnotherapy, building rapport is not just a tool or a technique; it is a skill which Brooks has perfected over many years. Building rapport goes far beyond the NLP techniques of matching body language and backtracking words. Body language is seen as a continuous expression of the unconscious mind and can be observed, mirrored, stimulated and utilised. The client's words are not simply backtracked but are shaped into indirect suggestions to depotentiate the conscious mind and encourage the unconscious. Furthermore, rapport building means not only tuning in to a client's thinking style, values, needs and beliefs but fully accepting and utilising these. Brooks' clients feel understood, valued and respected by him, even if they do not respect themselves. Rapport creates the basis for a client to feel safe, go into a trance, open up and take courage to change. For Brooks, it is not simply a principle to work from, it is a state of being he occupies from the moment of the first contact with the client.

Layered Approach

In many therapeutic orientations, information gathering, diagnosis and treatment occur linearly. First, the information is gathered, then the problem is diagnosed, then the therapy is performed. In Ericksonian hypnotherapy, however, the different stages greatly overlap or even merge together. Usually, a session begins with the gathering of some information about the client's problem and goal. At any point during this process, hypnotic induction or therapeutic intervention can start so trance can develop, symptoms can change, and more information can be gathered while this happens. Unconscious information becomes available and can immediately be used for trance deepening and further therapeutic suggestions. Trance phenomena can be used as a metaphor for the problem and for the solution. The experience of trance and any change in symptoms increases the client's trust in both the therapist and the therapeutic approach, allowing him to open up and reveal private information. In this way, information gathering, evoking trance, rapport building and therapy become one. The constituent elements are only differentiated for analysis or education.

Indirect communication

Milton Erickson was known for his extensive and artistic usage of indirect suggestion. It is one of the main characteristics that sets his work apart from traditional direct hypnosis. Brooks modelled this style of communication at the beginning of his career and soon excelled in it. Indirect communication includes the use of indirect language patterns, implication, presupposition, metaphor, analogy and symbolic tasking. Brooks combines all these elements in his highly condensed indirect communication style. Practically every sentence he utters is packed with indirect suggestions, implications and hidden messages. Indirect communication avoids or deflects resistance on the part of the client. It distracts, confuses or overloads the conscious mind, allowing the unconscious to express itself, to accept suggestions and to perform changes. Once rapport has been firmly established and the client is in a state of trance, with the conscious mind out of the way, Brooks will often switch to direct suggestion or, as he humorously puts it, "then I am going for the throat".

Confidence and Competence

In his teaching, Brooks emphasises the importance of confidence on the part of the therapist. Milton Erickson once stated:

> "Because my attitude towards my patients is: You are going to accomplish your purpose, your goal. And I am very confident. I look confident. I act confident. I speak in a confident way." (Zeig, 1980)

Brooks has that same level of confidence. It is expressed in his words, gestures, actions and general demeanour. Everything he says or does inspires confidence that he will be able to help the client and that the client will be able to help himself. This makes it easy for a client to trust him, to open up, to be receptive and to allow changes to happen. Even when he uses permissive, indirect or open-ended language, he acts and sounds confident. Every positive experience or therapeutic change during a session —and afterwards— increases the client's trust in him and in the therapy. A positive cycle of confidence and success is created, each contributing to the other. People who have been referred to him usually trust him even before meeting him; they expect to be healed and thereby greatly contribute to the success of the therapy. According to Brooks, new therapists must find the resources to feel confident, even though they may have little experience. This could mean taking confidence from success in other areas of their lives, activating positive past experiences, or visualising future successes. Confidence leads to success and successes increase confidence; this is a positive cycle that Brooks learned early in his career, and one that has increased his successes over the years.

Dedication, compassion and love

Closely related to the principle of rapport are the principles of dedication, compassion and love. Brooks considers these to be essential elements of great therapy. "The client is the most important person in my life at this moment," he often says. He will do whatever it takes for his client to make a change for the better. With this goal in mind, he is open, creative, flexible, bold and always prepared to try something new. Not only does he give the client suggestions, metaphors, tasks and experiences, he also gives him or her something of himself. This can be a present in the form of an object, a special word, even a hug. Sometimes he invites the client to take whatever he or she needs from him. Brooks has no fear of losing something of himself; he believes that the act of giving makes both the receiver and the giver richer. Giving love increases love on both sides.

Internal/external reality

In Ericksonian hypnotherapy and NLP, no representation or model of reality is true or fixed. Every person builds his own model of reality by gathering information and by having all kinds of experiences throughout his life. Every new experience is observed through lenses that are shaped by previous experience. People filter incoming information with these same lenses, focusing on certain things and excluding or ignoring others. An inner reality that works well and/or one that is shared with others is usually considered to be true. An unusual inner reality —e.g. seeing things that no one else can see— could be taken as a sign of mental illness or seen as a sign of creativity, even genius. Ericksonian hypnotherapy tends to tap into the latter. It uses trance to temporarily diminish or exclude external reality and explore the client's internal reality. In trance, this internal reality is expanded with trance phenomena like increased imagery, dissociation, automatism and hallucination; these phenomena help the client go beyond the usual logic and limitations. Hypnotherapy cannot change external reality, but it can change internal reality by changing perceptions, meanings, beliefs, thought processes and feelings. Brooks' approach helps people to open and expand their inner reality so that they can reach their personal goals and fulfil their dreams.

Process versus content

Brooks often says he is not interested in the content of the client's problem. He does not want to be drawn into the client's story and run the risk of believing in the client's perception. He gathers just enough information to understand the nature of the problem in order to know how to respond. Brooks focuses on process, not on content. In fact, a session can even be 'content-free', meaning that Brooks doesn't know what the client's problem is. He may simply bring the client into a trance and lead him or her in a positive direction by being artfully vague. On other occasions, the client may need to share what has happened, using the act of sharing as a way of relaxing and letting go. Generally, some content is beneficial to build rapport, to understand the client's ideas and feelings and to make the proper therapeutic choices. In the Spider Phobia session described in this book, Brooks gathers a little content information at the beginning before he starts a process of trance and therapeutic change.

Humour

Brooks uses humour in his sessions whenever he can. Even in sessions where the client is dealing with intense pain or sadness, he will introduce humour as soon as rapport is strong enough and a joke or pun might be helpful.[2] Part of Ericksonian hypnotherapy is to help the client step out of their problem and look at it objectively, take a different perspective. Quite often, people start laughing when they see the structure of their problem from the outside. They begin to see that their way of thinking and behaving is silly or even ridiculous. Brooks calls this "finding the fool in yourself"; in other words, it involves finding

---

[2] Humour can also contribute to rapport by showing the client that, not only can you understand and accept their perspective, you can also offer a very different one.

the part of you that has foolishly maintained the problem through limited ways of thinking and believing. Humour is also a way of overruling a negative state with a positive one. Needless to say, this principle only works when embedded within a firm basis of safety and trust.

Small change/big change

In Ericksonian hypnotherapy, it is believed that small, even minute, changes are significant in the process of growing and healing. Solving a cognitive, emotional, or social problem involves inner changes in perception, thinking and behaving. Clients frequently think they cannot make the big change that is required. For this reason, Brooks often breaks down the client's problem into the smallest possible components – to problems that are fairly easy to solve. This gives the client a sense of control and a means to bring about change. Milton Erickson sometimes suggested change in the 'wrong' direction, e.g. for an obese person to gain weight, simply to prove that change was possible. Another interesting hypnotic technique is to suggest a change that is so small that it is imperceptible to the conscious mind. This is a failsafe technique that involves change, whether or not the client notices it. Every change contributes to the client's confidence in taking the next step. He or she not only solves the current problem or situation but also learns the process of change. Brook's ambitious goal is not simply to help a client overcome a problem but to set up a generative process of change and healing that continues throughout the rest of his or her life.

Imagination/realisation

Walt Disney once stated, "If you can dream it, you can do it". This idea is at the heart of Brooks' work as a therapist. Whether the client wants to overcome an anxiety disorder, reach a professional goal or embark on a spiritual path, dreaming is a powerful way to make it happen. The state of trance allows the client access to the unconscious mind: the place where all dreams begin. The unconscious is momentarily freed from the limited and critical influence of the conscious and can create various images, sounds, ideas and feelings. In trance it is much easier to visualise and develop a flow of ideas and feelings; Brooks makes extensive use of this special state. He helps his clients to visualise their problems, fears and pains, either literally or metaphorically; in this way, the client gains control over them. He invites them to see, in their mind's eye, their goals, hopes, dreams and solutions as powerful motivators for change.

Chapter 2: Indirect Communication

Milton Erickson was famous for his various forms of indirect communication with a client. Ericksonian hypnotherapy is therefore known as indirect hypnotherapy because this 'indirectness' sets it apart from traditional (direct) hypnosis and from most other forms of psychotherapy. Brooks originally learned the art of indirect communication from Erickson but developed his own style which he has refined over the years. Like Erickson, he works indirectly whenever useful or necessary, and directly when possible. Direct communication is often more efficient when rapport is strong, and trance is deep enough for the client to be open and receptive. Brooks also uses direct suggestions if the client is accustomed to following orders or directives. He then simply matches the client's thinking style.

Indirect communication is effective whenever the client's conscious mind is proving obstructive and 'in the way', for example by analysing or evaluating the therapist's words and controlling unconscious responses. This is often the case in a first session, especially at the beginning. The client doesn't yet know the therapist and may not be familiar with hypnotherapy. You might say that he or she is 'on guard' and attempting to understand and control what happens. Indirect communication is a way of respecting this initial, conscious control, at the same time as inviting the client to start exploring unconscious thoughts, feelings, needs etc. When Brooks explains trance to the client, he is actually 'describing' what trance is to the conscious mind (satisfying it) while telling the unconscious to 'develop' it. For example:

> Hypnotic trance sometimes begins by experiencing *a certain heaviness in the eyelids.*

As soon as the unconscious responds to the embedded suggestion (a certain heaviness in the eyelids), the conscious mind begins to understand in an experiential way and can start to let go. Many therapists have difficulty leading their clients from thinking and talking about the problem to experiencing and feeling it. Direct instructions to stop thinking and start feeling often fail because the client doesn't feel understood or simply doesn't know how to do this. Indirect suggestion is an elegant way around this problem. If the client seems critical, sceptical or resistant, indirect communication is even more important. Here it can be used to distract, confuse or overload the critical, conscious mind and open the door for an unconscious process. An example of a confusing suggestion would be:

> I don't know if your *right hand* will become *light*, right away or your *left hand* will *lift* later.

The suggestions that the right or left hand may become light or lift are embedded in a slightly confusing sentence[3] designed to overload the conscious mind and get through to the unconscious.

Indirect communication is not restricted to hypnotherapy. In fact, indirect language is used in everyday life, although not always effectively. The simple question "Can you pass me the sugar?" is an indirect way of saying "Pass me the sugar". "I wonder how you feel" is an indirect way of asking "How do you feel?" Some people have learned to talk indirectly so well that they have difficulty asking direct questions or uttering direct statements. A young child's language is still direct as a child has not yet learned to communicate indirectly. Parents are often embarrassed by the very direct statements their children make in public. As a child grows older, he or she learns that people do not always appreciate direct words. The child begins to understand that others might feel offended, insulted or even attacked when thoughts are expressed directly. Children intuitively learn to abstract, wrap up or sugar-coat their messages in order to get their meaning across, reach their goal or keep the peace.

The level of indirectness and abstraction varies widely depending on culture, life experience, education, beliefs, values and profession. Politicians, managers and salespeople are often creatively indirect in delivering their messages. Surgeons, firefighters, childcare workers and members of many other such professions have to be direct in order to reach their communication goals. In Ericksonian hypnotherapy, indirect communication is key for distracting the conscious mind to reach the unconscious. Brooks has taken this to the highest level and turned indirect speech into an art form. When he communicates in an artfully vague

3 The rhyme (right/light) and alliteration (left/lift/later) are additional appeals to the unconscious.

and indirect way, his clients rarely show resistance to his questions, ideas or suggestions. They are quickly guided towards their unconscious resources and solutions. As a result, his therapy is usually brief and successful. In this chapter, we describe the various forms of indirect communication —originating from the work of Milton Erickson— used by Brooks in the Spider Phobia session that is described in Part 2 of this book.

Embedded suggestions

With embedded suggestions[4], the actual suggestion is embedded (hidden) in a larger sentence or story. Usually, the embedded suggestion is marked out — for example, with a different voice tone. While the conscious mind is busy processing the entire sentence, the unconscious mind can pick up on the marked, embedded suggestion.

People use embedded suggestions all the time in everyday situations, usually without being aware of doing so. If you want somebody to give you a certain object —a key, for example— you might say, "*Give me the key*". This would be a direct suggestion. If you wanted to be more indirect, you could say, "Can you *give me the key*?", "*Give me the key*, please" or "I want you to *give me the key*". All these sentences can have a slightly different effect on the listener. The extra words distract, please or satisfy the conscious mind so that it does not control the more or less automatic (unconscious) response of handing over the key. Therapeutic suggestions are often much less concrete than the above example. Usually, they are suggestions about ideas, feelings, behaviours or beliefs. The direct suggestion to "*feel relaxed*" might cause resistance in the client. He or she might consciously think, "I don't know how". The indirect suggestion "I wonder how long it will take for you to *feel relaxed*" contains the same message, but it is hidden in a fairly complex sentence. Conscious attention is drawn to the therapist's thinking (I wonder) and the amount of time required (how long it will take) and away from the actual suggestion (feel relaxed). Slightly emphasising (analogue marking) the words *feel relaxed* has the added effect of alerting the unconscious to the suggestion. Any word, phrase, sentence or story can be used to embed a suggestion, as long as it keeps the conscious mind busy. There are, however, special language structures that not only embed a suggestion but add

[4] Embedded suggestions are also known as embedded commands.

extra meaning or turn the suggestion into a presupposition. In this chapter, we will describe the language structures Brooks uses to embed suggestions in the Spider Phobia session.

Sentence adverbs

Adverbs are words that qualify verbs, adjectives or other adverbs. In the sentence "I totally understand what you mean", the adverb 'totally' qualifies the verb 'understand'. Sentence adverbs are slightly more complex because they qualify an entire sentence or clause. They are often words ending with 'ly', like: 'actually', 'clearly', 'probably', 'certainly', 'gradually', 'usually', 'generally', 'normally' and 'fortunately'. Other examples are the words: 'nevertheless', 'therefore', 'perhaps', 'however', 'indeed', 'also', 'maybe' and the phrases 'as such' and 'in fact'. Sentence adverbs turn the phrase that follows into an embedded suggestion or embedded statement. Some examples are:

> <u>Actually,</u> *this is easy to solve.*
>
> <u>Certainly,</u> *this will change.*
>
> <u>Clearly,</u> *you can do something about it.*
>
> <u>Interestingly</u>, many people with this problem *have overcome it.*
>
> <u>In fact</u>, *the process of healing is completely natural.*

Sentence adverbs momentarily distract the conscious mind, just long enough for the unconscious to absorb the embedded suggestion. Although they often come at the beginning of a clause, they can also be used in the middle or at the end:

> <u>Actually,</u> *this is easy to solve.*
>
> *This is,* <u>actually</u>, *easy to solve.*
>
> *This is easy to solve,* <u>actually</u>.

The function of a sentence adverb is not just to entertain the conscious mind. It also tells the unconscious mind how to understand the suggestion that follows. The adverb 'certainly' has a different connotation to 'probably', which in turn is different to 'maybe'. Brooks chooses his adverbs carefully to pace or lead the client. Pacing means choosing words that match the client's vocabulary, beliefs or thinking style. To a client who uses the word 'actually' a lot, you can say:

> <u>Actually</u>, *trance is a wonderful experience.*

The conscious mind will easily accept the word 'actually' as familiar and, the unconscious can pick up its meaning ('really'). So, while satisfying the conscious, we are telling the unconscious to create a 'really wonderful trance'. To a client who thinks in terms of black and white we could say:

Certainly, we will go for a complete *resolution of this problem.*

To a client who is very hesitant about starting hypnotherapy, we can say:

Maybe we can take a first step towards *solving your problem.*

Examples from the Spider Phobia session:

What you have is fairly common, actually.

You experience, maybe, *some fluttering.*

In fact, *they look prettier with them open than with them closed.*

Time adverbs

Time adverbs are adverbs that refer to the time or frequency of an event, state or action. They are words like 'now', 'then', 'in a moment', 'in the future', 'sometimes', 'often',[5] etc. Often, they appear at the beginning of a sentence:

In a moment, you can *go into trance.*

Sometimes, it is nice to *go into trance.*

Now, you can begin to *discover all kinds of resources.*

Each time you are here, *you will discover something interesting.*

Sometimes, they are used in the middle or at the end of a sentence:

You can, now, *go into trance.*

You can *go into trance* now.

How these time adverbs are received and processed by the client depends on the way they are delivered. The therapist can direct the adverb[6] 'in a moment' to the conscious mind and the suggestion *you can go into trance* to the unconscious mind,

[5] Note that words like 'now' and then refer to points in time whereas 'sometimes' and 'often' refer to frequency.

[6] Actually, 'in a moment' is an adverbial phrase, rather than an adverb.

using analogue marking. The conscious mind can process the time predicate whereas the unconscious can (immediately) follow the suggestion.

In a moment... *you can go into trance.*

Alternatively, the therapist can direct the entire sentence to the unconscious mind (no analogue marking).

In a moment you can go into trance.

The unconscious mind is instructed to delay the trance 'for a moment'. Obviously, 'a moment' is a vague term and the unconscious can still choose how long that will be. Brooks often uses the word 'now' in his communication. Used at the beginning of a sentence, the word 'now' can be a time adverb used to orient the client to the present moment. Sometimes, however, it is a discourse marker (see below), similar to words like 'okay' and 'so'; used in this manner, it is a word that connects the suggestion to whatever was said before. Depending on the previous sentence, the position of the word 'now', and the use of emphases and pauses, 'now' can have different functions.

Just allow your arm to relax ... now (now = this moment)

You were lonely back then. Now, you have friends. (now = nowadays)

Now, can I ask you something? (discourse marker)

Besides using time adverbs, suggestions can be embedded with place adverbs like: here, there, somewhere, anywhere, nearby and outside. For example:

Here *you can explore all your resources.*

Somewhere *you will find the answer to your question.*

Brooks often uses a combination of time and place adverbs. For example:

As you are here now you can *go into a state of relaxation*

Examples from the Spider Phobia session:

Then, as *your arm starts to get heavy, you go a little deeper relaxed.*

Each time you breathe out, *a little deeper relaxed.*

As you lie on the beach, here now, just to *find a cloud.*

Now, *say on and watch it go on* again.

Now here I'd like you to *start to move towards your own body.*

In a moment, I'm going to count to three, when I reach the number three, the harder you *try to bend that arm*, the more *rigid it becomes.*

Degree adverbs

Degree adverbs are adverbs that refer to the extent or degree of a state, process or action. They are words like 'just', 'too', 'almost', 'very', 'hardly', 'deeply', 'absolutely'. They can be used at the beginning of a sentence, before an actual suggestion:

Just *tell me what is on your mind.*

Simply *try it out and see what happens.*

As such, an imperative sentence (a command) is embedded in and softened with a single word. Brooks often uses the word 'just' this way. This single word not only makes the command indirect but it also suggests it is easy to execute. A variation of this is the use of 'just' in a sentence fragment with the verb in the gerund form. For example:

Just *letting go.*

Obviously, degree adverbs can also appear within a suggestion rather than before it. For example:

You can be deeply relaxed.

Here the adverb is not used to embed the suggestion but to qualify a state or process and turn it into a presupposition (see chapter 4).

Examples from the Spider Phobia session:

Just *relax every muscle.*

Just *allow yourself to float up out of your body.*

Just *going deeper relaxed.*

Just *relaxing and hear the sound of my voice.*

Qualifying adjectives

Another way to make a suggestion indirect is to use the structure:

"it is <adjective> to" or "it is <adjective> that"

Qualifying adjectives are used here, like: easy, interesting, imaginable, good, funny, nice, possible or strange. For example:

It is easy to *go into trance.*[7]

It is imaginable that *you can let this go.*

It is interesting to *experience hypnosis.*

Embedded suggestions like this can also take the form "it is a <adjective> <noun> to" or "it is a <adjective> <noun> that":

It is an easy task to *go into trance.*

It is an interesting idea that *you can let this go.*

Sometimes, qualifying adjectives are used in conjunction with the gerund (e.g. knowing) rather than the infinitive (to know):

It is fantastic knowing you can relax.

Like sentence adverbs described previously, qualifying adjectives can be carefully chosen to pace or lead the client's thinking or behaviour.

Examples from the Spider Phobia session:

Notice how easy it has been *taking things a step at a time.*

As you see, it might be interesting for you to *hear that.*

How nice to be able to *do that*, just enjoy being on the beach now.

Noun phrase

Yet another way to make an embedded suggestion is to use the introductory structure "the <noun> is to…" where <noun> is a nominalisation. For example:

The idea is to *use hypnosis to help you achieve your goals.*

The plan is to *discover the best way for you to go into trance.*

Your role is to *simply be here and allow these changes to occur.*

---

[7] This is the same as "*to go into trance* is easy" but with the to-clause extra posed to the end of the sentence.

A variation on this structure is "the <noun> is that..." or "the <noun> of/to/about... is that...". For example:

> <u>The advantage is that</u> *you can learn from experience.*
>
> <u>The result of this step is that</u> *you can be yourself from now on.*

Examples from the Spider Phobia session:

> <u>The wonderful thing about this is that</u> *it's all yours.*
>
> Now <u>her job is to</u> *make him feel comfortable and not scared.*

Verbs of thinking and feeling

These are verbs that express someone's mental or emotional state or activity. Examples are: 'to think', 'to feel', 'to expect', 'to trust', 'to forget', 'to decide', 'to regret', 'to be aware', 'to be sorry'. In Ericksonian hypnotherapy, they can be used to make a suggestion or statement indirect. For example:

> <u>I think</u> *you can achieve your goals.*
>
> <u>You can trust</u> that *your problem can be solved.*
>
> <u>I feel</u> *you already have what it takes.*
>
> <u>You know</u> *you can go into a deep trance.*

Some verbs of thinking and feeling, like 'to know' and 'to realise' are so-called factive verbs. They not only embed the suggestion that follows, they also presuppose it (see chapter 4).

Examples from the Spider Phobia session:

> *He feels a bit embarrassed* <u>I think</u>.
>
> <u>She feels herself</u> as if *she is a projected baby.*
>
> <u>I know</u>, with the laser, *you can write with a laser.*
>
> (I am) <u>sorry</u> *I am so much bigger than you.*

Embedded questions

Embedded questions are questions that are inserted into statements [8]. Such statements start with phrases like: 'I wonder', 'I don't know', 'I ask myself' and 'I'm curious'. For example:

> I don't know if you have experienced hypnotherapy before.
>
>> Embedded question: Have you experienced hypnotherapy before?
>
> I was wondering whether this problem also occurs at home.
>
>> Embedded question: Does this problem also occur at home?
>
> I am curious about what you have learned about yourself.
>
>> Embedded question: What have you learned about yourself?
>
> I ask myself how *I can help you.*
>
>> Embedded question: How can I help you?
>>
>> Embedded suggestion: *I can help you.*

Note that the first three examples are indirect requests for information, whereas the last one is actually an indirect suggestion. In Ericksonian hypnotherapy, the lines between information gathering and influencing are deliberately blurred and, questions often act as suggestions.

Embedded questions can refer to the therapist or to the client. In the latter case, they are often used with a modal operator like 'can' or 'might'.

> You might ask yourself when the problem doesn't occur.
>
>> Embedded question: When doesn't the problem occur?
>
> You can wonder how *this problem will be solved.*
>
>> Embedded question: How will this problem be solved?
>> Embedded suggestion: *This problem will be solved.*
>
> You may be curious about when *this change will occur spontaneously.*
>
>> Embedded question: when will this change occur spontaneously?

---

[8] They can also be included in larger questions, e.g.: "Can you tell me *when this first started*?"

Embedded suggestion: *this change will occur spontaneously.*

Apart from making a suggestion indirect, embedded questions encourage a state of curiosity, which is usually helpful in problem-solving.

Examples from the Spider Phobia session:

> And you can wonder whether you *go all the way down, into a nice deep comfortable, relaxed state.*
>
> And you might wonder how you knew, how a *part of you knew, that your eyelids had to flutter to help you experience this.*

Modal operators

Modal operators are verbs that change the modus of another verb. 'Can' is a frequently used modal operator for making a suggestion indirect. Some examples:

> You can *go into trance.*
>
> Can you *go into trance*?

The suggestion to *go into trance* is embedded in the phrase 'you can' or 'can you'. The conscious mind is alerted to the 'ability' of going into trance rather than the 'behaviour' of doing so. The question in the second example is also called a conversational postulate. This is a question which grammatically requires a yes or no answer but is usually received as a request or suggestion. There are modal operators of:

> Possibility: can, be able to, may
>
> Necessity: must, should, have to
>
> Desirability: want to, need to, like to
>
> Choice: choose to, select, decide to

Modal operators do not necessarily create embedded suggestions; they can also be part of a direct suggestion or statement. Suppose a client has doubts about his ability to go into trance, the hypnotherapist might say:

> You *can go into trance.*

Stressing the word 'can', would then be a direct statement about the client's trance-ability. Brooks uses modal operators in both ways; to embed a suggestion or to suggest a possibility or ability.

Clients use modal operators as a part of their language patterns, often without being aware of it. Many people create stress in their daily lives by excessive use of modal operators of necessity. They might say or think things like:

> I have to finish this project today.
>
> I should control my emotions.

Others limit their experience by using negative modal operators of possibility. They use sentences like:

> I can't make a decision.
>
> I cannot be assertive.

Here, modal operators are not used to create embedded suggestions but rather act as limiting beliefs. When you hear modal operators like these in your client's story, you can utilise them to induce trance or offer therapy. For example:

> It is interesting to notice that you can't open your eyes, isn't it?

Not being able to open your eyes is a trance phenomenon (eye catalepsy) and a powerful convincer of hypnosis. This way, you use the client's negative linguistic patterns to their own advantage, which is the essence of utilisation. On the other hand, you can lead a client away from using limiting modal operators like 'have to' and 'can't' to supporting operators like 'can', 'want to' and 'choose to'.

Examples from the Spider Phobia session:

> You can *learn to recognise something.*
>
> I'd like you, to notice that, you can *go very, very deeply relaxed.*
>
> What you should do, is *look at him and tell him that you'll find him again.*
>
> And this is something that may *surprise you.*
>
> She decides to *make it a friend*, to *become friends with it.*
>
> Now you can *feel comfortable and confident and happy with any insects.*

Discourse markers

A discourse marker is a word that marks a piece or segment of verbal communication. It connects the upcoming statement or suggestion to the previous communication or to the wider context. Examples are words like 'so', 'now', 'well', 'okay', 'oh', 'and', 'but', 'or', 'so', 'anyway' and 'because'. As well as word combinations like: 'I mean', and 'you know'. One characteristic of discourse markers is that they can be omitted without changing the meaning of the rest of the sentence. They do, however, serve a useful linguistic purpose: they provide a certain structure and cohesion in a conversation (Schiffrin, 1987). They can also be used as a minimal form of embedding suggestions; usually with a single word. Discourse markers often appear at the beginning of a statement, suggestion or question. For example:

> <u>So</u>, hypnosis is a powerful way to change your life.
>
> <u>Now</u>, take a deep breath.
>
> <u>I mean</u>, do you really want to go on like this?

The conscious mind will assess the meaning of the discourse marker and the relation it suggests between what was said (or what happened) before and what follows. The unconscious mind can then pick up the idea or suggestion that follows. Sometimes a discourse marker appears at the end of a sentence. For example:

> Going into trance is easy, <u>you know</u>.

The words that are used as discourse markers can also belong to other categories: 'and', 'or', 'but' and 'so' can be used as conjunctions; 'now' can be used as a time adverb; and 'you know' can be used as a factive verb. The category a certain word belongs to depends on its position, linguistic environment, and pronunciation[9].

> <u>You **know**</u> *this can be solved.*
>
> Factive verb because the word **know** is emphasised.
>
> <u>Y'know,</u> ....*this can be solved.*

---

[9] The criteria for words to be assigned as discourse markers as well as role of discourse markers is rather complex and beyond the scope of this book. For a detailed description of discourse markers see (Schiffrin, 1987)

Discourse marker because 'you know' is contracted to 'y'know', it is not emphasised, and it is followed by a pause.

This can be solved y'know.

Discourse marker because it is contracted and appears after the actual statement.

Now, *that was easy.*

The word 'now' is a discourse marker here. It cannot be a time adverb (meaning the present moment) because that would conflict with the word 'was' (past tense).

Now *that is easy.*

Time adverb because the word 'now' is emphasised and does not conflict with the word 'is' (present tense).

I invite the reader to recite the above sentences several times, varying the pronunciation of the word 'now' and the phrases 'you know' and 'y'know'. You may use voice tone, emphasis, volume, pitch, pauses or even try stretching out the word 'now'. Brooks often uses ambiguous pronunciations, leaving it to the client to interpret his words. The grammatical function of any word is primarily relevant for analysis or education. What matters in a session is the way in which the client understands our words and utilises them to change his or her experience and thinking.

Examples from the Spider Phobia session:

You can *learn to recognise something,* y'know.

So, because it is a learned thing, *we can change it very easily.*

Well, you know *you can project things on this cloud.*

Because *she's gonna be very relaxed on the beach.*

Okay, what I'd like you to do is *watch the cloud kind of get misty.*

Now, notice how *easy it has been, a step at a time.*

Explicit requests

People have many ways of suggesting or requesting others to do something. If, for example, someone is smoking in a non-smoking area and you want him or her to stop, you can do that directly or indirectly, implicitly or explicitly. For example:

> Implicit suggestion: You are smoking in a non-smoking area.
>
> Explicit direct suggestion: *Stop smoking here.*
>
> Explicit and embedded suggestion: It is a good idea to *stop smoking here.*
>
> Explicit and embedded request: I want you to *stop smoking here.*

The difference between the last two examples is that the latter explicitly states the speaker's wish. Instead of 'I want you to' more subtle expressions like 'I would like you to' and 'please' can be used. Hypnotherapeutic examples might be:

> I want you to *go into trance.*
>
> I would like you to *take a deep breath.*
>
> Please, *tell me all about it.*

Brooks uses this form of suggestion; not to force his will upon a client, but rather to take a strong leading position with a client who would benefit from it.

Although the explicit request sounds like a very direct form of suggestion, it is actually indirect because the conscious mind is directed toward the therapist's wish (I want you to…) while the unconscious mind can process the embedded suggestion (go into trance). The level of indirectness can be influenced by analogue marking. The more the actual suggestion (go into trance) is separated from the embedding phrase, the more indirect it becomes.

Examples from the Spider Phobia session:

> I'd like you to notice that you can *go very, very deeply relaxed.*
>
> What I want you to experience, as you *keep your eye on that ring there.*
>
> When *it starts to lower,* I want you to *go deeply and deeply relaxed.*
>
> I want you to *allow, allow, the laser to write the letter P.*

Announcement

Another way of rendering a suggestion or statement indirect is by announcing it before giving it. People often use them in daily life when they have something unpleasant or upsetting to tell you; for example, "I need to tell you something. I have wrecked your car." Here the entire suggestion consists of two complete sentences. Examples within the hypnotherapeutic practice could be:

> I'll tell you what you can do. You can practise this until you know you can do it.
>
> I have a request for you. Stand up and stretch out your hands now.
>
> I am going to ask you a question. What does this all mean to you?
>
> I want to tell you a story. When I was a little boy...

Announcing a suggestion makes it indirect and also creates curiosity and expectancy. The longer the pause between the announcement and the actual suggestion, the more curious, expectant or even frustrated the client will become.

Announcements like these can be used for a suggestion but also for a question, request, or story. The experienced difference between the explicit request described in the previous paragraph and the announcement becomes clear in the following examples:

> Explicit request: I want you to *put both feet on the ground.*
>
> Announcement: I want you to do something. *Put both feet on the ground.*

The announcement contains the vague word 'something'. If you use a brief pause between the announcement and the actual suggestion, the conscious mind can wonder what 'something' means and wait for specification, while the unconscious can immediately translate 'something' to specific ideas or actions. So, after the actual suggestion, the client might *put both feet on the ground* and do other relevant things.

Announcements can also occur in a one-sentence form using the verb *going to* (or *gonna*). For example:

> You are going to *experience something new.*
>
> We are gonna *solve this problem.*

In daily life, these kind statements are used to express ideas about the future: expectations, predictions, plans, etc. For example: "you are going to have a good time" or "we are gonna get married". In hypnotherapy, this structure can also be used to create an embedded suggestion. The conscious can understand and accept the entire sentence as an idea for the future whereas the unconscious can (immediately) execute the embedded suggestion.

Examples from the Spider Phobia session are:

> Now, a story. *<name client> just told me...*
>
> You are going to *feel more relaxed* than you have for a long time.
>
> I'd like you to learn something else. And that is that *you can float up, out of your body.*

Linguistic softeners

The use of linguistic softeners is a subtle way of softening or reducing a suggestion or statement. Words and phrases like 'almost', 'kind of' and 'as if' create this effect.

> You can almost *see the solution.*
>
> Now, you can kind of *see that in your mind's eye.*

Also, Brooks frequently uses the combination of 'almost' and 'as if', as in one of the examples from the Spider Phobia session:

> I would like you to, kind of *collect your thoughts.*
>
> *They will become rigid,* almost as if *there is an iron bar inside.*

Quotes

Quotation is yet another form of indirect communication. The people who are being quoted are not usually in the room, so it is harder to resist their opinion. Furthermore, you can characterise the quoted person as intelligent, experienced, benevolent etc. to increase the power of your message. The source of a quote can be specific, or it can be vague.

Specific source

Here the person who is quoted is specified.

> My father used to say to me: *you can do whatever you want.*
>
> Stephen Brooks always says: *trance is glue that makes suggestions stick.*

Some clients draw on important or famous people as a source of information. Quoting such people will help those clients accept your suggestion.

Einstein said: *imagination is more important than logic.*

Milton Erickson said: *The unconscious works without your knowledge, and that is the way it prefers.* (Erickson & Rossi, 1980c)

Unspecified source

It is not always necessary to specify the source of a quote. The fact that you are quoting somebody is enough for many clients, and it still makes your suggestion indirect, for example:

Someone once told me: *he was surprised how deeply he could go into trance.*

A famous therapist once said: *The curious paradox is that when I accept myself just as I am, then I can change.*

Extended quote

Quoting a single line, once said by somebody, usually renders a suggestion indirect enough to circumvent the conscious mind. Some clients, however, are very analytical and 'see through' this trick. They realise that it is actually 'you' saying it to them. If you expect this to happen, you can hide your message in an extended quote. Here you quote someone who, in turn, cites someone else. For example:

"I recently ran into a friend of mine who told me about his boss telling him he had *every reason to be proud of himself.*"

Obviously, a suggestion can be hidden even more deeply in a longer story or metaphor where someone quotes someone else who quotes a third person etc.

Tags

Tags are grammatical structures that turn a statement or command into a question. In Ericksonian hypnotherapy, they are used to anticipate or deflect possible negation by the client and to encourage agreement. Some examples:

You can *go into a trance*, can you not?

It is nice, to *feel relaxed*, isn't it?

Things will improve, will they not?

Note that the second suggestion (feel relaxed) is made indirect with a qualifying adjective (It is nice) and with a tag (isn't it). A combination of these forms would be:

> Isn't it nice, to *feel relaxed*?

The two forms have the same elements but offer different opportunities for analogue marking; they will therefore have a different effect on the client. Brooks is keenly aware of each of these variations and their possible impact. He constantly observes his client while talking, adapting his words, voice tone, emphasis and use of pauses to the client´s minimal cues and other non-verbal responses.

Examples from the Spider Phobia session are:

> *You know what the word is*, do you not?
>
> How do you feel looking up at that word? *You feel okay*, do you not?
>
> *Feels pretty neutral*, doesn't it?
>
> Don't you, want to *help that little thing*?

Using the client's name

Expressing the client's name encourages him or her to take a suggestion as personal. Besides analogue marking, it is another way of alerting the unconscious mind to an embedded suggestion. The pattern is often used in combination with a modal operator, like 'can'. The name of the client can be inserted at various positions in the sentence and, each position will create a different effect.

> You can *go into trance.*
>
> John, you can *go into trance.*
>
> You can, John, *go into trance.*
>
> You can *go into trance*, John.

In the first example, the client can apply the suggestion to himself (I can go into trance) or to people in general (one can go into trance). In the second example, he can only apply it to himself (I can go into trance). Still, it is a permissive suggestion. In the third example, his name is placed between the modal operator 'can' and the actual suggestion. As such, the latter acts as a direct suggestion or command (go into trance). In the last example, the client has the freedom of applying the suggestion to himself or to people in general, until his name is mentioned. Then he must apply it to himself. By playing with the position and intonation of the client's name —as well as using pauses— a suggestion can be made less or more direct or personal. A few other examples, not using 'can' as the modal operator are:

> Some people want to, John, *go into trance.*
>
> It is interesting to, John, *go into trance.*

Examples from the Spider Phobia session:

> And while you are doing that, <name client>, I'm going to talk.

Embedded statements

So far, we have discussed embedded suggestions: suggestions about something that the client can do, think or feel. However, a statement or a description can also be embedded in a sentence to similar effect. Where suggestions are used to stimulate the client to do something (mentally or behaviourally), statements are often used to make the client learn or understand something.

Note the difference between:

> Embedded suggestion: It is interesting to *go into trance.*
>
> Embedded statement: It is interesting that *trance happens all by itself.*

Both are using the qualifying adjective (it is interesting) to make the rest of the sentence indirect. In the first case, it is 'suggested' the client go into trance; in the second, the client is 'informed' that trance happens all by itself. In hypnotherapy suggestion and statement greatly overlap and embedded statements, or parts of them, often act as embedded suggestions. Usually, they are statements (information) for the conscious mind and suggestions for the unconscious mind.

> It is good, to know, that hypnosis can help you to *overcome your fear.*
>
> Are you aware, that you are *in a trance right now?*
>
> Sometimes, people *go into trance* easily.

Examples from the Spider Phobia session:

> So see *what you have is fairly common* actually.

So *they are quite special* in fact, aren't they?

You know *things have already started to change.*

After all, *it's a harmless thing.*

Negative embedded suggestions

Here a suggestion is embedded in words with a negative connotation. You can use words like 'not', 'difficult', 'impossible', or 'undesirable'. For example:

It is rather difficult to *go into trance.*

You can't *go into trance.*

I don't want you to *go into trance.*

Nobody told you to *go into trance.*

Just like using tags, this is a way of pacing or deflecting negative beliefs, attitudes or expectations. The conscious mind can agree to the negative statement (yes, it is difficult) as the unconscious follows the suggestion (go into trance). Here's how it works: if the client agrees (yes, it is difficult), the conscious mind is engaged in a yes-set while the unconscious starts to develop trance. If the client disagrees (no, it's not difficult), the conscious is now engaged contradicting the therapist and actually, supporting the unconscious in following the suggestion by going into trance. Rapport is still maintained because the client will probably not argue with the therapist but will enjoy proving him wrong. It's like saying to a child, "I bet you can't eat this big sandwich". The child will enjoy proving you wrong, and you can give praise and compliments when they do. With these negative statements, clients often find themselves in a double bind: whether they agree or not, they will tend to follow the suggestion.

If you want to use the above suggestions in a subtler way you might say:

You would think it would be rather difficult to *go into trance.*

So it seems you can't *go into trance.*

I don't want you to *go into trance*, just yet.

Who told you to *go into trance?*

These too, pace the client's negative beliefs, but they do it more indirectly. Furthermore, these suggestions imply the opposite of what they are saying. 'It seems you can't' implies 'you actually can', especially if the word 'seems' is emphasised.

Examples from the Spider Phobia session:

> But it's gonna be difficult to *see what it is.*
>
> She can't *make out what it is at first.*
>
> It can't *get out of the cloud.*
>
> *Maybe* you can't quite *see his face*, at the moment.

Multiple embedded suggestions

Obviously, the more complex the linguistic structure of the embedded suggestion, the more tied up the conscious mind becomes and the easier it is for the suggestion to reach the unconscious. Consider the suggestion '*go into trance*', as part of an increasingly complex and increasingly indirect suggestion:

> *Go into trance.*
>
> Now *go into trance*
>
> You can *go into trance.*
>
> When will you *go into trance?*
>
> I wonder when you will *go into trance.*
>
> Then she said to me you can *go into trance.*
>
> I wonder when you will realise that you can *go into trance.*
>
> Then she said to me I wonder when you will realise that you can *go into trance*, isn't that interesting.

Note that in the last example, the actual suggestion is wrapped up in five statements, four before and one after the actual message. In a regular conversation, a sentence like that might seem artificial and overcomplex. But in therapy —especially in hypnotherapy— it can be used to overload the conscious mind or to build curiosity and expectation. By the time the actual suggestion is given, the conscious mind is completely tied up and confused. Brooks skillfully uses words, phrases, voice tones, pauses, gestures and facial expressions to mark and shape various parts of his sentences. He offers his messages to the client in a complex and condensed verbal/nonverbal package, and he constantly adapts his language to the client's style and development. Although highly complex, the conversation seems casual and natural to the client.

There are many words or phrases that can be used to create embedded suggestions. In general, however, we want to limit ourselves to words that are familiar to our clients or that they find acceptable, interesting or maybe confusing. The type of indirect communication that works best for a particular client depends on his or her thinking style, beliefs and values. Those familiar with NLP meta-programs (thinking styles), can use the model to help tailor their indirect communication to suit their clients. For example:

> Meta-programs: 'internal reference' and 'options':
>
> > You know, there are many ways, to *go into trance.*
>
> Meta-programs: 'external reference' and 'procedure':
>
> > I know, there are a number of steps you can follow, to *go into trance.*
>
> Meta-program: 'polarity response':
>
> > Don't *go into trance.*
>
> Meta-program: 'in-time'
>
> > I wonder how it feels for you to *go into trance* now.
>
> Meta-program: 'through-time'
>
> > I wonder how you can see yourself *go into trance* in the course of time.

Interspersal technique

The interspersal technique is similar to embedded suggestions in the sense that a message is hidden in a larger linguistic structure. It was developed by Milton Erickson, who used it with clients who were particularly sceptical about hypnosis or therapy (Erickson & Rossi, 1979) (Erickson & Rossi, 1980b). With the interspersal technique, suggestions, ideas or messages are interwoven in a story, analogy or intervention. The story is seemingly unrelated to the client's problem but must be acceptable, interesting or captivating for the conscious mind. Meanwhile the unconscious can pick up and absorb the interspersed ideas. If, for example, you want to introduce the idea of freedom to a client, you could use an embedded suggestion like:

> I wonder when you will start to *feel freedom.*

Or I could tell a story:

> I was walking on the beach the other day, enjoying the sound of the ocean and the warmth of the sun. When I looked up I saw a bird high in the sky and imagined the sense of *freedom* a bird *can feel* just being up there. I realised where the expression *'free as a bird'* comes from.

Obviously, the interspersed idea is even more indirect than the embedded suggestion. In both cases, analogue marking is used to alert the unconscious to the idea of interest. Milton Erickson sometimes used interspersal as the main technique in a session. He would engage the client in a long metaphor or analogy during which he would repeat an idea in various forms. Brooks often uses metaphors or analogies as a part of a session, alongside trance induction and therapeutic intervention. At the start of a session he uses stories to seed ideas or elicit states; later he uses them to develop and solidify those ideas or states and transfer them to the future. At the beginning of the Spider Phobia session, Brooks intersperses the idea of 'learning' and 'unlearning'. States of 'relaxation', 'comfort' and 'dissociation' are interspersed throughout, and in the latter part, notions of 'trust' and 'friendship' are interspersed.

Talking to others

Milton Erickson occasionally talked to someone other than the client to make his communication indirect. He would, for example, hypnotise someone else in the room in order to indirectly hypnotise the client. Or he would talk to a different person and use embedded suggestions to direct specific parts of that communication to the client. In education and Play Therapy, this technique is used by talking to a doll to deliver a message to a child. Brooks often uses this form of communication in his demonstrations in front of live audiences. Before, during or after the session he will turn to the audience and explain aspects of his dialogue with the client. Certain parts of this explanation, however, are suggestions for the client. He will casually turn his face and direct his voice to the client while saying these words, and then turn back to the audience. In fact, this communication technique has two goals: it is an explanation to the audience (overt goal) and a suggestion to the client (covert goal). I (JvB) use this technique in training courses or in my practice when a partner, parent or friend of the client is present. I will say things to the other person or ask them questions while observing how my client responds. Indirect suggestions of trance presented as an explanation to an audience could be:

> <u>As I will demonstrate to you all</u>, *trance happens all by itself.*
>
> <u>In a minute I am going to show you how quickly someone can</u> *go into trance.*

In the Spider Phobia session, Brooks uses the technique of talking to others at the beginning of the session. He explains the idea of scaling the problem between 0 and 10 to the audience and concludes with the suggestion, "We are going to bring that right down". Towards the end of the session, Brooks again addresses the audience, saying:

> "I guarantee that she will use it anyway because *this worked*, and she's gonna see *it worked.*"

He briefly turns his head in the client's direction when he says *this worked.*

Analogue marking

This is the technique of nonverbally 'marking' certain parts of a sentence or story using voice pitch, volume or tonality, voice direction, gaze direction, facial expression, postures, gestures or pauses. In doing this, the actual suggestion stands out from the rest of the sentence and is easily picked up by the unconscious. Suggestions using voice tone might be:

> You know, there are many ways, to ***go into trance.***
>
> Isn't it nice, to ***feel relaxed?***

When multiple suggestions are communicated, say during trance inductions and therapeutic interventions, or when telling metaphors and analogies, the hypnotherapist can repeat a certain form of analogue marking for a certain experience. He can, for example, use a soft voice each time he wants the client to go deeper in trance. He can direct his voice upwards each time he talks to the conscious mind and downwards when he talks to the unconscious. As a form of visual marking, he can open his hands whenever he invites the client to open up. When talking to people other than the client, the main form of analogue marking is voice direction. If the analogue marking is used consistently, it is not just a way of emphasising something; it becomes a way of anchoring a certain response to a certain signal. It is worth noting that it's not only the hypnotherapist who uses analogue marking; clients use it too, to emphasise parts of their message or elicit a certain response in the therapist. The difference is that clients are not usually aware that they are doing this whereas hypnotherapists do it deliberately.

Brooks uses analogue marking all the time. He plays with his voice and varies his body language to highlight certain syllables, words, phrases or sentences. Obviously, it makes a difference depending on whether the client's eyes are open or closed. With eyes open, the client can see the therapist's facial expressions, gestures or changes in posture. As soon as the eyes close, these visual signals disappear, and auditory marking becomes more important. Despite this, Brooks uses posture, gestures, and movement when the client's eyes are closed because he is convinced that his movements influence his voice and can be sensed by the client. With his background as a musician and 40 years' experience as a therapist, he is highly skilled in moving and influencing people with his words, voice, and body language. His use of analogue marking is an art more than a technique.

Chapter 3: Being Artfully Vague

A special form of being indirect is the use of vague language. In everyday life, vague language might be regarded as a negative thing. Politicians, for example, are often accused of being vague and challenged to speak in more concrete or specific terms. In hypnotherapy, however, vague language is considered something positive. Milton Erickson used a myriad of vague language constructions to pace and lead his clients. He referred to this communication style as 'being artfully vague'. A large part of Ericksonian hypnotherapy consists of the creative and intelligent usage of vague language.

Before we tackle vague language, let's have a look at language in general. People use it for various purposes: to express themselves, to make contact, to inform, and to amuse or comfort others. On the other hand, it can be used to insult, control or manipulate. Language can be a powerful tool, and it can be a lethal weapon. Verbal communication can take place in the form of questions, statements or commands. Language can be direct or indirect, concrete or vague.

Using vague and indirect language is a skill that people acquire over the years. When a child begins to use actual words, these are usually concrete nouns: the names of observable objects like parts of the body, toys, pets and people. The child uses words like 'hand', 'nose', 'mum', 'dad', 'dog', 'bottle' etc. Later, he or she learns to use concrete verbs, which describe observable events, behaviours and actions: words like 'eat', 'drink', 'walk' etc. A young child's thoughts are concrete representations of things and actions from the outside world in the form of images, sounds and feelings. His or her language consists of words referring to those representations. The child lives in a concrete world. Later, he or she begins to develop the skill of abstraction: the ability to think of things that are not directly observable. The child learns to understand and talk about concepts, ideas, categories and processes. He or she acquires words that refer to things that exist only in the mind, not in the outer world. Objects and actions are no longer simply observed and named; they are also interpreted, evaluated and judged. Words like 'good', 'bad', 'okay', 'nice', 'naughty', 'ugly' and 'beautiful', become part of the child's vocabulary. Objects are grouped into categories. Doll, ball and puzzle all belong to the category 'toys'. The child becomes aware of the concept of time and learns the words referring to it; 'now', 'later', 'tomorrow', 'in a minute', 'at 9 o'clock' etc. The concept of counting is taught and words like 'one', 'two', 'hundred', 'few' and 'many' are acquired. The child learns the idea of negation; something that is 'not' there or 'should not' be there. He or she starts to understand messages like "the doll is *gone*" and "*don't* touch that". The child also learns about the consequences of certain actions (real or imaginary) from warnings like "If you yell at her, she will be scared". For a new-born baby, nothing has meaning; a baby observes with all of its senses and responds instinctively. Part of education is learning about meaning: the meaning of things and actions. Meaning only exists in the human mind; it does not exist in the world. It is, by definition, imaginary, although people often experience the meaning of something as being very real. Meaning, interpretation and categorisation make our thinking and language abstract. Our choice of study and profession will strongly influence the level of abstraction we acquire. A baker, mechanic, surgeon, or hairdresser will probably need to think and talk in much more specific terms than a teacher, songwriter, manager or politician.

There are many reasons for using vague language: communicating with large groups of people, summarising a story, hiding specific information or influencing others. Politicians excel in the use of vague language in order to get their messages to the widest possible audience and to make it difficult for anyone to hold them to account for lying or breaking promises. Poets and songwriters use vague language creatively to entertain people or touch their hearts. Hypnotherapists use vague language to pace their client's experience and lead it in a positive direction. When a client hears vague words, he or she will automatically translate them into concrete images, sounds and feelings. This is the only way to make sense of vague language. With positive vague suggestions, the client is nudged in a therapeutic direction, while having the freedom to create his or her own personal experience. Resistance is avoided because nothing is said that could contradict the client's reality. Brooks has learned the artistry of vague language (mainly from Erickson's work), practised it over many years and taken it to a new level of sophistication. This chapter gives you a list of vague language constructions as he uses them with his clients.

Nominalisations

A nominalisation is the result of turning a predicate —i.e. a verb— into a noun. Nominalising a verb means freezing an action or process in time and turning it into an abstract thing. Nominalisations refer to ideas, concepts, or categories (e.g. respect, failure, mankind) rather than to objects or matter (e.g. pencil, chair, water). A nominalisation is, by definition, vague and means different things to different people. The phrase "respect is important" does not inform the listener who is supposed to respect whom or when, where and how this should happen. This is all left to the imagination of the listener. Nominalisations can have a positive, negative, or neutral connotation depending on the listener's understanding of the word. They play an important role in Ericksonian hypnotherapy to pace the client's current experience and lead it into his or her desired direction. Brooks makes extensive use of nominalisations in his work with clients.

Negative nominalisations

Negatively-charged nominalisations are used to pace the client's negative experience and, as such, to build rapport. Brooks might pick up a certain word from the client's language, or sense that a certain word fits his or her experience. Negatively-charged nominalisations are words like:

> problem, crisis, depression, addiction, difficulty, trouble, blockage, burden, pain, stress, symptom, danger, hell, fight

Examples from the Spider Phobia session:

> severity, tension, illness, phobia, problem, severity, tension, worry, problem

Apart from pacing the client's experience, negative nominalisations can also be used to challenge or provoke, e.g. "Sounds like absolute hell to me". Typically, clients will play down such a statement with something along the lines of "Well, it's not that bad"; in doing so, they assert themselves and look at the problem from a more positive perspective. The field of Provocative Therapy is based on this principle. Although Brooks is not a provocative therapist, he uses this principle whenever he considers it useful.

Positive nominalisations

Positive nominalisations are those with a positive connotation. They are used to lead the client's experience in a desired, positive direction. These are words like:

safety, choice, love, balance, experience, excitement, surprise, trance, understanding, ability, strengths, power, discovery, courage, pleasure, connection

Examples from the Spider Phobia session:

help, change, freedom, warmth, control, respect, adventure, community, gift

To understand these words, the client has to create a representation of them. By hearing and representing the word 'change', he or she will, at some level, experience it. Even if he or she consciously thinks, "I don't how to change", the change might take place on an unconscious level. As Bandler and Grinder noted:

> "In order to understand what I mean when I say the word 'relax', you have to go inside and access your personal experiences related to that word. You have a fragment of the experience as a way of understanding the word itself." (Bandler & Grinder, 1981)

Neutral nominalisations

Nominalisations with a neutral connotation can be used to either pace or lead the client's experience. These are words like:

situation, thought, process, path, emotion, idea, experience, journey

Examples from the Spider Phobia session:

thing, way, memory, situation, question, scale, idea, illustration, reference, demonstration, moment, state, experience, distance, step

Obviously, any nominalisation can be positive for one person but neutral or negative for another. The question is always, "What does a certain word mean to the client?"

To understand nominalisations more deeply, let's have a closer look at their origin. Many nominalisations are derived from the corresponding verbs. For example, the words 'failure', 'development' and 'solution' are derived from the (vague) verbs 'to fail', 'to develop' and 'to solve', respectively. Other nominalisations come from their corresponding adjectives. For example: sadness, possibility, and wisdom come from the adjectives sad, possible and wise. Some nominalisations stem from predicates in foreign languages. The word 'crisis' comes from the Greek word 'krisis', meaning decision, so it's actually a nominalisation of the verb 'to decide'. The word 'hypno' (as in hypnosis and hypnotherapy) comes from the Greek word 'hypnos', meaning sleep, a nominalisation of the verb 'to sleep'. Although some nominalisations are derived from the adjectives, the reverse also exists. Various adjectives/adverbs are derived from nominalisations. Words like 'dangerous(ly)', 'miraculous(ly)', 'painful(ly)', 'beautiful(ly)' and 'delightful(ly)' come from the nominalisations: 'danger', 'miracle', 'pain', 'beauty' and 'delight'. For example:

> ...and now you can let go of those painful feelings and start enjoying that miraculous sensation of joy.

Actually, the linguistic source of a certain nominalisation is not that important, as long as you realise that it is a vague noun that your client will translate to a concrete representation. The classic NLP trick to distinguish a nominalisation from a concrete noun is to ask oneself, "Can I put it in a wheelbarrow?" [10] Now, a 'shoe' can be put in a wheelbarrow, but a 'solution' cannot. Therefore, the word solution is a nominalisation.

Brooks has a talent for using the right nominalisations; i.e. the ones that match the client's experience or need. He might use a certain word because:

- it was expressed by the client, and he wants to feed it back to him or her
- it matches the client's nonverbal cues
- it matches the client's background, lifestyle, profession or age
- it is general enough to fit most people (like *problem* and *solution*)

His choice of words is probably based on a mixture of these criteria. He says he often isn't aware of the origin of his verbal expressions. After years of experience and thousands of sessions, he is unconsciously competent in using vague language and tailoring it to the client's needs. A nominalisation is not right or wrong of its own virtue. It is the effect it has on the client that determines its value. As I (JvB) often say to my students, "More important than saying the right things is observing the effect of what you say and utilising that".

---

10 The wheelbarrow can be as big as it needs to be, e.g. to hold a house, a plane, or even a planet.

Vague verbs

Vague verbs are verbs that refer to conceptual processes rather than observable activities. As with nominalisations, vague verbs mean different things to different people. They can have a negative, neutral or positive connotation and they can be used to pace or lead the client's experience.

Negative vague verbs

Vague verbs with a negative connotation are used to pace (or challenge) the client's negative experience. These are words like:

> to hesitate, to block, to disturb, to hide, to lose, to insult, to disrespect, to ignore, to hate

Examples from the Spider Phobia session:

> to scream, to hurt, to frighten, to panic, to kill, to worry

Positive vague verbs

Brooks uses vague verbs with positive connotations to lead the client's experience in a positive direction. These are words like:

> to solve, to delight, to free, to let go, to accept, to value, to respect, to love, to cherish, to celebrate, to control

Examples from the Spider Phobia session:

> to learn, to surprise, to manage, to help, to achieve, to congratulate, to free, to play, to smile, to trust, to please, to relax

Neutral vague verbs

Vague verbs with a neutral connotation can be used to either pace or lead the client's experience. These are words like:

> to discover, to experience, to find, to let go, to change, to enter

Examples from the Spider Phobia session:

> to happen, to bring, to meet, to work, to drift, to imagine, to happen, to project, to absorb, to fade, to experience, to discover, to realise, to become

Obviously, any vague verb can be positive for one person and negative for another.

Vague adjectives and adverbs

Adjectives and adverbs play an important role in everyday language and in hypnotic language. Adjectives qualify nouns, which, in hypnotherapy, are often nominalisations.

> "You can have an *exciting* journey."

The word 'exciting' not only influences the client's interpretation of the word journey, it will create its own representation. The greater the emphasis on the word 'exciting' and the longer the pause after it, the more the client will start to think of specific exciting 'things'.

Adverbs qualify verbs [11] which in hypnotherapy are often vague verbs.

> "You can *easily* develop that skill."

Some adjectives are derived from nominalisations, for example, 'beautiful' and 'dangerous'. Others come from vague verbs, for example, 'interesting' and 'acceptable'. Adjectives and adverbs are often vague, although some are vaguer than others. A 'wonderful trance' is vaguer than a 'deep trance' because 'deep' only refers to the depth aspect of the trance whereas 'wonderful' can refer to any aspect.

Negative adjectives/adverbs

Vague adjectives and adverbs with a negative connotation are used to pace (or challenge) the client's negative experience. These are words like:

> Adjectives: blocking, disturbing, bad, frightening, hateful, negative, terrible.
>
> Adverbs: terribly, disturbingly, hopelessly, cruelly, neurotically, obsessively.

Examples from the Spider Phobia session:

> Adjectives: bad, hard, nasty, difficult, scared.

---

[11] or adjectives or other adverbs.

Adverbs: badly.

Positive vague adjectives

Brooks uses vague adjectives with positive connotations to lead the client's experience in a positive direction. These are words like:

> Adjective: delightful, brave, acceptable, valuable, good, nice, loving, creative, fantastic.
>
> Adverbs: delightfully, beautifully, gently, naturally, well, better, near.

Examples from the Spider Phobia session:

> Adjectives: harmless, good, easy, strong, confident, special, nice, relaxed, delighted, lovely, wonderful, peaceful, convenient, grateful, excited, happy, beautiful.
>
> Adverbs: luckily, fully, perfectly, deeply, automatically, easily, comfortably.

Many adjectives and adverbs such as real/really and constant/constantly are in themselves neutral. It is the linguistic context and the client's interpretation that makes them positive, negative or neutral.

> Now you can *really* relax.
>
> I am in *constant* pain.
>
> Maybe you need some *tough* love.

Did you realise that the word 'nominalisation' is a nominalisation itself, that 'specific' and 'vague' are both vague adjectives and that 'specifically' and 'vaguely' are vague adverbs? Is your conscious mind getting somewhat confused? Good, because as Milton Erickson used to say, "enlightenment is always preceded by confusion".

Loaded words

These are vague words that carry a lot of personal, cultural or spiritual meaning. They can be categorised as emotive or high-inference, and include words like 'secret', 'miracle', 'ultimate', 'peace', 'love', 'victory', 'seduce', 'severe', 'terror', 'hell', 'enemy' and 'horrible'. They can be nouns (nominalisations), verbs, adjectives or adverbs and they can have a positive or negative connotation. In marketing, loaded words are used to attach meaning and emotion to products and to evoke a wish or need to buy them, in consumers. In politics, they are often used to influence potential voters or denigrate opponents. In hypnotherapy loaded words are used to elicit unconscious emotions, needs, memories or resources. They can also be applied to create surprise or shock.

Examples from the spider phobia session are:

> perfectly, freedom, to surprise, delighted, to dream, to transform, community, fool, crazy, incredible, hypnosis, gift.

Unspecified reference

Another way of being artfully vague is by using unspecified references. These can be references to 'people', 'places', 'times' or 'objects'. Words like 'someone', 'somewhere', 'sometime' and 'something' are vague; they don't give any specifics about the 'who', 'where', 'when' or 'what'. To understand these words, the listener will have to make them specific in his or her own mind.

Unspecified person

Instead of talking about the client or someone in the client's life, a reference to an unspecified person can be used. This leaves the client the freedom of applying the message to herself or not. References to an unspecified person or persons include words like 'we', 'one', 'people', 'they', 'someone'. Here are some examples with embedded suggestions:

> Some people go into trance by closing their eyes.
>
> Often friends are more supportive than you expect.

The word 'you' can be used as a specific reference (you the client), or as an unspecific reference (anybody), depending on voice tone and emphasis.

> Sometimes, **you** don't know where the answer comes from.
>
> Sometimes, you don't **know** where the answer comes from.

In the first example, the word 'you' refers to the client (actually to the client's conscious mind) whereas in the second example it refers to people in general.

Examples from the Spider Phobia session:

> Who could she become? Someone else or something else?

You know what happens when you call people by name.

Unspecified time

Instead of suggesting specific times or timeframes, unspecified references can be used. Now, the client has the freedom to apply the suggestion to any moment in time or any life stage. Unspecified references to time are words like 'someday', 'any moment', 'soon', 'recently',' long ago', 'in the old days', 'in your childhood', 'in little a while'. Some example suggestions are:

> Soon, you will *go into a comfortable trance.*
>
> Someday, *things will start to change.*
>
> A lot of *things happened* in your childhood.

Note that the degree of vagueness or specificity of the words varies. For example, 'when you were young', 'in your childhood' and 'in your school days' are all vague references to time, but they are increasingly specific. Some vague references refer to the past (e.g. 'recently') while others refer to the future (e.g. 'soon'). Even references to the present may vary in specificity; 'in this day and age', 'nowadays', 'now', 'right now', 'this second', are all vague references to the present, but they are increasingly specific.

Examples from the Spider Phobia session:

> The moment *she is lying on the beach looking up at the cloud.*
>
> If you think at any time she could feel uncomfortable, just *say the word 'off'.*
>
> And she's gonna thank you later, for *helping her achieve this* as well.
>
> Because in the past she knew what it felt like to be scared of something.

Unspecified place

Instead of mentioning a concrete location or context, unspecified references to place can be used. This allows the client the freedom to apply the message to any place or context in his or her life (including none). Unspecified references to place are words like 'somewhere', 'over there', 'in a certain place', 'far from here', 'nearby' etc. For example:

> Just pick a spot over there and focus on it.

I am sure the answer is somewhere out there waiting for you.

Examples from the Spider Phobia session:

> If you were somewhere *very comfortable and special*, like on a holiday or somewhere you know is a very nice place to be.
>
> And the wonderful thing about this is that it's all yours, this special place.
>
> Now, I'd like you to find somewhere convenient, to *rest that cloud*, somewhere on the ground, somewhere, just *rest the cloud*, somewhere, somewhere convenient. Not too far away, nearby.

In this last example, Brooks goes back and forth between being totally vague (somewhere, not too far away) and a little more specific (somewhere on the ground, nearby).

Unspecified object/event

To reference an unspecified object, we use a vague word referring to a thing (physical or conceptual). Examples: 'something', 'things', 'a process', 'an event'.

> Something will happen after you open your eyes.
>
> As you know, things change all the time.

Note that references to unspecified objects are nominalisations. In fact, they are very vague nominalisations; they say only that 'something' exists but give no information about what it is.

Examples from the Spider Phobia session:

> Because in the past she knew what it felt like to be scared of something.
>
> And this is something that may surprise you.

Unspecified process

Unspecified processes are words that refer to the nature, process or way of things. These are words like 'somehow', 'in some way', 'one way or the other', 'along a certain path' and 'like that'.

> Somehow you can *go into trance.*
>
> One way or the other your unconscious will *help you in achieving your goal.*

Again, it is left to the client to go on an internal search for specificity, to see, hear or feel specific ways of going into trance or achieving his or her goal.

Note that the unspecified reference 'somehow' is also a sentence adverb (see Chapter 2) that turns the rest of the sentence into an embedded suggestion. This is a nice example of the combination of vague and indirect language.

Examples from the Spider Phobia session:

> Be aware of your arm in the air like that.
>
> And somehow it looks friendlier.
>
> Because somehow you feel drawn towards that cloud.

Comparative deletion

In a comparative deletion, words implying a comparison are used, but the standard or reference is omitted. You compare someone or something but, you don't say with whom or with what. Comparisons can be created with words like 'different', 'the same', 'comparable', 'similar' etc. They can also arise from the use of the comparative/superlative form of adjectives like 'big/bigger/biggest', 'bright/brighter/brightest', 'good/better/best'.

> Going into trance is a different experience.
>
> It is much easier to relax.
>
> That is the greatest challenge.

None of these examples specify the reference for comparison. The client will unconsciously search for a reference to answer the inevitable questions, "different to what?", "easier than what/when/where?" and "greatest within which list or category?"

Examples from the Spider Phobia session:

> Just deeper relaxed, each time you breathe out.
>
> Now you can bring it lower bring it down lower.
>
> So it gets a little bit bigger. A little bit closer.
>
> It's not the same one, it's a different cloud.
>
> The best gifts are the ones that you don't actually get appreciation for.

Lost performative

Brooks often uses statements expressing certain assumptions or beliefs without specifying their reference or origin. They can be quotes, sayings, general expressions or even modified versions of clients' negative beliefs. The vagueness involved here is that of 'lost performative' because the person who first expressed the statement (the performer) is not mentioned. Statements with lost performative aren't necessarily true, but when they are nicely embedded and expressed with confidence, they are likely to be accepted by the client. A client with an external reference might consider the statement to be an expression of the therapist's wisdom. For example:

> Life isn't about finding yourself. Life is about creating yourself.
>
> > A quote from George Bernard Shaw.
>
> Practice makes perfect.
>
> > A proverb.
>
> Overcoming a depression takes time.
>
> > A modification of a client's belief "Overcoming my depression will take a long time."

The first example is a vague statement with lost performative if the quoted person is not mentioned. If he is mentioned, however, it becomes an embedded vague statement [12] (see Chapter 2):

> George Bernard Shaw once said: "Life isn't about finding yourself. Life is about *creating yourself*."

Examples from the Spider Phobia session:

> It's always important to *have a good family*

Using articles

In the grammar of hypnotic language, articles are used to create the illusion of specificity in a sentence that is actually vague. Note the difference between the sentences:

---

[12] A statement with the embedded suggestion '*creating yourself*.

An experience that will change your life.

The experience that will change your life

That experience that will change your life.

They only differ in the article of the word 'experience': indefinite (an), definite (the) or demonstrative (that). With each successive sentence, there is an increasing suggestion of specificity. This may be easier to see when the articles are used with a concrete object:

Take a pen.

Take the pen.

Take that pen.

Anyone who understands English will intuitively understand the implications in these sentences. The first sentence simply implies that one or more pens exist. The second one implies that there is a special pen (or just one pen) and that both the speaker and the listener know that. The third sentence implies that one or more (depending on whether or not the word that is emphasised) pens are available but that one pen is being referred to.

In a regular conversation, these implications are usually true. If someone says to you, "Please give me *that* pen", he might be pointing to a certain pen or refer to a pen that was mentioned before. If there is no pen, the request will not make much sense. In Ericksonian hypnotherapy, we can use the definite (the) or demonstrative (that) article without referring to anything specific. We can say, "you know you have *that* quality" with no specific quality in mind. This is possible because we use nominalisations rather than concrete objects. Nominalisations are realised in the mind; they do not exist in the outer world. As a hypnotherapist, you can talk about '*the* experience' or '*that* development' without specifying or even knowing what you mean. The client will find or create his or her own representations of these words. Although you may not know what you mean by '*that* quality', the client might believe that you do. He or she can assume that you see a special quality, perhaps one that he or she is not aware of. If the client (the conscious mind) asks which quality you mean, you could simply answer:

"I wonder when your unconscious mind will let you know what quality *that* is."

This response will shift the responsibility for answering the question from you to the client's unconscious, and it allows you to repeat the suggestion that he or she has '*that* quality'. Skilful usage of various articles is yet another way of being artfully vague.

Examples from the Spider Phobia session:

> But <u>that</u> movement and the fluttering in your eyelids is so characteristic of a good hypnotic subject.
>
> Just be of aware of <u>that</u> warmth in your head.
>
> Let it write <u>the</u> word.
>
> And as <u>that</u> image or picture starts to form, I want you to watch her, because she's gonna be very relaxed on the beach, totally relaxed and confident and comfortable.

Universal quantifiers

Universal quantifiers are generalisations of 'person', 'time', 'place', or 'object' that include all members or no members. These are words like 'everyone', 'always', 'everywhere', 'everything' and 'nobody', 'never', 'nowhere', and 'nothing'. They are similar to unspecified references like 'someone', 'sometime', 'somewhere' and 'something', but take it to the extreme. As unspecified references, universal quantifiers leave it up to the client to make the translation to specific people, times, places and things. The use of universals makes a suggestion more dramatic.

Including all members

Universal quantifiers including all members are words like 'everyone', 'always', 'everywhere', 'everything' or words with a similar meaning.

> <u>Everybody</u> knows *you can do it.*
>
> <u>Every person in the world</u> has a right to *live happily.*
>
> People *go into trance*, <u>anywhere</u> around the world.
>
> These resources have <u>always</u> been there, waiting to be used.

Everything happens for a reason.

Examples from the Spider Phobia session:

You will always *be very very confident.*

Just *relax* every muscle, every muscle, anytime I touch you on the shoulder here.

If you take things a step at a time, almost anything is possible.

And you didn't know that all around you, if you look hard enough, you can *find a bunch of wonderful friends.*

Now you can *feel comfortable and confident and happy* with any insects.

Don't they always tell you something those eyes?

Excluding all members

Universal quantifiers excluding all members are words like 'nobody', 'never', 'nowhere', and 'nothing', or words with a similar meaning.

Nobody can keep you from *going into trance.*

There was never a better moment for you to *take this step*, was there?

There is no place you can't go.

Nothing stands in the way of our goal.

Not a single thing will hold you back.

Examples from the Spider Phobia session:

Once you are confident with spiders, you will never ever go back to how it used to be.

And that child will never know about it, never realise what you gave it back here.

Universal quantifiers are generalisations. On a conscious level, the client might agree or disagree with them. In either case, he or she will unconsciously make it specific and create the corresponding experience. In response to the statement, "Everyone knows you can do it", the client might consciously think, "No, not everyone" while visualising people who don't. However, the implication of defining some people who don't know is that others 'do' know and the unconscious picks up on that implication. Or the client might think, "That's true, everyone does know that" while visualising specific people who do. The result at the unconscious level is the same: a specific representation of people who know that he or she can do it.

Universal quantifiers work well with clients who tend to generalise and use universals themselves. They usually find it easy to consciously accept the suggestion and unconsciously represent it. People who are 'matchers'[13] will respond better to universals including all members.

> You know you can <u>always</u> feel good about who you are, <u>anywhere on earth</u>.

People who are 'mismatchers' might respond better to universals excluding all members.

> I want you to realise that <u>nobody</u> can <u>ever</u> take that away from you.

Meta-programs (thinking styles) like matching/mismatching are context-dependent and can change during the course of therapy. If your client seems to have a mixed style —or if you are not sure about his or her thinking style— you can simply use both kinds of universal:

> You can <u>always</u> be relaxed, you'll <u>never</u> have to be tense anymore.

Brooks uses universals, not just to be vague, but also to make a suggestion more intense. He does this by adding certain degree adverbs (like absolutely, entirely, completely) and by emphasising the universal quantifier:

> There is <u>**absolutely nothing**</u> that can keep you from being happy.

Omitting the personal pronoun

As described before, the personal pronoun of a sentence (usually 'you' when addressing the client) can be replaced by an unspecified or universal reference. As such, the client is not directly addressed and has the freedom to apply the suggestion to him or herself or not. A third option for indirectly addressing the

13 An NLP meta-program: matchers focus on things that are present, correct or good whereas mismatchers focus on things that are missing, incorrect or bad.

client is to remove the personal pronoun altogether. Consider the following suggestions:

> *You* can go into trance (specific)
>
> *People* can go into trance (unspecified reference)
>
> *Everyone* can go into trance (universal quantifier)
>
> *Going into trance* is easy (no personal pronoun)

The last example contains no personal pronoun and has the phrase "going into trance" as a subject. There are several ways of avoiding the use of a personal pronoun in a sentence or phrase. The trick is to replace them with nouns, verbs that act as nouns or dummy subjects, or as Brooks often does, use the gerund in an incomplete sentence.

Nominalisations (vague nouns)

> Trance is a gateway to the unconscious.
>
> Energy flows where attention goes.

Gerund phrase as noun

> Going into trance can be a pleasant experience.
>
> The good thing about experiencing this, is that it can change.
>
> It is a question of letting go.

Infinitive phrase as noun

> To go into trance is easy.
>
> It is easy to go into trance. [14]
>
> It is not difficult to explore this.
>
> It is a good idea to change that pattern.

Dummy subject

> There are many pathways to this goal.

---

[14] Here the actual subject "to go into trance" is extraposed to the end and replaced by an anticipatory *it.*

Actually, there is only one way to find out.

It is well known that there is always another chance.

Gerund in an incomplete sentence

Doing very well.

Just going deeper relaxed.

In none of the above statements is the client addressed. Most clients will not be aware of this and will automatically apply the suggestion to themselves.

Examples from the Spider Phobia session:

Congratulations on getting here now.

It is just a question of learning.

Just going deeper relaxed.

There's one more step to go.

Permissive language

A very common way of being vague —familiar to most therapists and intuitively used by many people— is permissive language. Here we talk about words like 'maybe', 'perhaps' and 'possibly'. Some examples are:

Perhaps, *you will go into trance.*

Maybe *that will start to lift.*

Permissive language also comprises the use of modal operators such as 'can', 'may', 'could' and 'might'.

You can *go into trance* at any moment.

You might *experience some differences.*

Permissive language allows the client the freedom to follow the given suggestion or not. He or she cannot fail because the suggestion was given as a possibility and not as a necessity.

Students of Ericksonian hypnotherapy sometimes argue that the client might interpret permissive language as doubt or insecurity on the part of the therapist. If, however, the suggestion is delivered with confident body language and voice tone, this is usually not a problem. When expressed from a position of confidence, permissive language can be both open and powerful.

Examples from the Spider Phobia session:

> You can let your mind wander.
>
> As you experience maybe some fluttering in your eyelids, some movements in your eyelids, realise that that fluttering and moving in your eyelids can help you, with your problem, you might wonder how that can happen.

Open-ended suggestion

Open-ended suggestions do exactly what the name implies; they suggest that something will happen, but what this will be, and how, when and where it will occur is left open.

> You can just be here and wonder what will happen.
>
> Hypnotic trance can happen in various ways.
>
> And you can take any step to sort this out.

Examples from the Spider Phobia session:

> They always say, you know, if you take things a step at a time, almost anything is possible.

As an alternative to leaving thing completely open, Brooks sometimes suggests a few specific options and then adds a general one. An example of this technique is:

> You can experience the lightness or heaviness in those hands or any other kind of sensation.

The client is invited to focus on the weight of his or her hands and at the same time permitted to experience any other feelings.

Examples from the Spider Phobia session:

> If you were somewhere very comfortable and special, like on a holiday or somewhere you know is a very nice place to be.
>
> He knows that she won't suddenly stamp on him, or do anything dramatic.

I want you to just...in your mind…you think of the spider or anything like that.

Covering all possibilities of a class

This pattern is similar to open-ended suggestions. The difference is that the hypnotherapist now sums up all possible options within a certain class. For example:

> You can go into a light trance, a medium trance, or a deep trance.
>
> You can bring that image closer or move it farther away.
>
> Which hand is the heaviest, the right one or the left one?

To make sure everything is covered, you can mention various specific options and add a vague one:

> I wonder if that hand will go up or down or in a different direction.
>
> You know that fear might vanish slowly or quickly or exactly at its own speed.

Alternatively, you can suggest another option without actually mentioning it, leaving an ungrammatical sentence:

> You can go into trance with your eyes open or closed or...

Sometimes you might want to offer all the possible options of a class but promote a specific one. This can be useful if the unconscious has already let you know it favours a certain option, and you want to acknowledge this. Let's say you saw the right-hand move slightly upwards a few times. You can offer two options for hand levitation while marking out one of them:

> Which one will lift, the left one or the **right one**?

If this analogue marking is done subtly enough, the client will experience the right-hand lifting without knowing why.[15]

Examples from the Spider Phobia session:

---

15 In daily life people can emphasise one of the options they offer, based on their own beliefs, wishes or possibilities, often without realising it. Obviously, this is something a hypnotherapist should avoid.

And you can be in the sun or in the shade, it is entirely up to you.

Some cloud up there, and is it to your left or to your right?

Is it on the ground yet, or is it still up in the air?

Ambiguity

When we talk about nominalisations, vague verbs, or vague adjective/adverbs, we are talking about words with one meaning, albeit a vague one. The word 'courage', for example, has one meaning that can be experienced and expressed in many ways. The word 'vision', however, has different meanings for example, 'the ability to see' or 'something seen in a dream or trance'. Likewise, the word 'solution' has two meanings: 'the process or result of solving a problem' and 'the result of dissolving a substance in a liquid'. The word 'light' can refer to weight or to illumination. The words 'vision', 'solution' and 'light' are examples of ambiguous nominalisations. [16] The words 'here' and 'hear' sound the same but have entirely different meanings. Language can be ambiguous in many ways including sound, syntax, scope or punctuation. In hypnotherapy, we use ambiguity to confuse the conscious mind and offer multiple options to the unconscious. Let's have a look at some forms of ambiguity that Brooks uses with his clients.

Phonological ambiguity

Phonological ambiguity refers to words that sound the same but have different meanings. We can distinguish homonyms, which are spelt and pronounced the same, and homophones, which only sound the same.

Homonyms

Homonyms are words with multiple meanings. An example is the word 'light', which can be the opposite of dark or darkness or the opposite of heavy. Another example is 'rose', which can be a flower or the past tense of the verb 'to rise'.

Soon, it will get *lighter.*

[16] Note that the word *vision* has two different but related meanings, whereas *solution* and *light* have different and unrelated meanings.

Used to enhance arm levitation (your arm will get lighter) and/or problem resolution (your burden will get lighter).

You know that on the *right* side, things will change.

Used to suggest changes on the right (right-hand) side of the body and/or problem resolution (on the positive side of your life).

Examples from the Spider Phobia session:

We are going to bring that right down.

Here it comes, little legs going right crazy.

Homophones

These are words that sound the same but are spelt differently and have a different grammatical form. Examples are: I/eye, here/hear, no/know, read/red, knows/nose, not/knot, to/too/two, in security/insecurity, transformation/trance formation, ahead/a head, your/you're. Note that with some homophones, one form consists of one word whereas the other consists of two words (transformation/trance formation). A homophone that is often used in Ericksonian hypnotherapy is wonder/wander. Although not exactly the same sound they are close enough to be confusing.[17]

Now you can take the time to wonder/wander...

It invites the client to consciously wonder, maybe about resources, possibilities and solutions and unconsciously wander, in time and in the world. Another one is:

You can trust your/you're unconscious now.

This can mean "you can trust *your unconscious* now" or "you can trust….*you're unconscious* now". The second meaning leaves it up to the client whom or what he or she can trust, and suggests unconscious functioning (you are unconscious). A slight pause after the word 'trust' and a subtle change of tone can emphasise the second meaning.

Homophones are sometimes used in incomplete or ill-formed sentences:

---

17 Also the therapist's pronunciation of the word can be deliberately ambiguous.

This is important to/too...

This can be interpreted as the complete sentence "This is important too" or the incomplete sentence "This is important to..." If you emphasise the last word and pronounce it with a slightly higher pitch, the client will probably hear it as 'too' and experience it as a complete sentence. If it is pronounced in the same tone as the word 'important', the client will hear it as 'to' and finish the incomplete sentence in his or her own head. With an ambiguous pronunciation, the client can be confused (consciously) and pick the most suitable form (unconsciously).

Homophones are also used in ill-formed, run-on sentences with punctuation ambiguities. Some examples are:

> You are here/hear the sound of my voice.
>
> It is important to know/no one can do this alone.
>
> You can go ahead/a head full of ideas.
>
> You're right/your right hand can start to lift.

You will find more about the punctuation ambiguity below.

Examples from the Spider Phobia session:

> You can let your mind wonder/wander around the beach.
>
> Maybe hear/here the sound of the sea.
>
> Just relaxing and here/hear the sound of my voice.
>
> The next thing for you to do is to spend some time wondering/wandering around the corridors here.

Syntactic ambiguity

Here the syntactic function of a word is unclear. The standard format is:

> <transitive verb>+ing <noun plural>, can[18] be <adjective>

This sentence is ambiguous because the transitive verb can also serve as an adjective. The classic example from the world of hypnosis is:

> Hypnotising hypnotists can be tricky.

---

[18] Or another modal operator like *may*.

This could mean: 'It can be tricky to hypnotise a hypnotist', or 'It can be tricky when a hypnotist hypnotises somebody'. Note that if you replace 'can be' with 'is' or 'are', the sentence is no longer ambiguous. An example for trance induction:

Lifting hands can be fascinating.

or therapy:

Changing minds can be interesting.

An example —often used by Milton Erickson— with a somewhat different format is:

The feeling of the chair.

Here it is unclear if this means "the client is feeling the chair" or "the chair has a feeling".

Scope ambiguity

In scope ambiguities, a phrase applies to another part of the sentence, but it is unclear which part.

Pleasant thoughts and feelings...

It is unclear if the adjective pleasant refers to 'thoughts and feelings' or only to 'thoughts'.

Do you realise that change is already occurring and trance is developing?

It is unclear if the phrase 'do you realise' only refers to the 'occurring changes' or also to the 'developing trance'.

A sentence often used by Milton Erickson is:

Speaking to you as a child. (Bandler & Grinder, 1975)

It is unclear if 'as a child' refers to the speaker or to the listener.

Examples from the Spider Phobia session:

Very comfortable and relaxed.

Punctuation ambiguity

With punctuation ambiguities, two well-formed sentences overlap to give one ill-formed run-on sentence. An example for trance induction:

> You can go into trance happens all by itself.
>
> > Here, an ill-formed sentence is constructed from the well-formed sentences 'you can go into trance' and 'trance happens all by itself'.
>
> Those worries are leaving you relaxed and secure.
>
> > A combination of 'those worries are leaving you' and 'leaving you relaxed and secure'.
>
> You are here/hear the sound my voice.
>
> > A homophone used to combine 'you are here' and 'hear the sound of my voice'.
>
> You're right/your right hand can start to lift.
>
> > A homophone used to combine 'you're right' and 'your right hand can lift'.

Ill-formed sentences are automatically corrected and therefore repeated by the client.

Examples from the Spider Phobia session:

> You can let your mind wonder/wander around the beach.

Chunking

In NLP, the term 'chunking' is used for changing the level of abstraction. Chunking up means moving to higher abstractions (vaguer), chunking down means moving to lower abstractions (more specific) and lateral chunking refers to moving on the same level of abstraction. In the following example, drawn from the physical world, the human body is a high chunk while the arm and head are two smaller chunks of the body. Finally, the hand and elbow are two smaller chunks of arm.

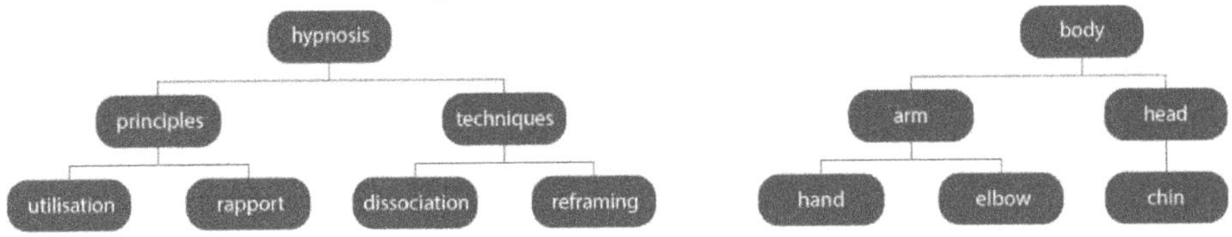

An example in the conceptual world would be 'hypnosis' as a high chunk, 'principles' and 'techniques' as two smaller chunks and 'utilisation' and 'rapport' as two smaller chunks of principles. Big chunks are categories, values, meanings, processes, identities, whereas small chunks are specific objects, actions, images, or physical feelings. Clients often use negative vague terms (high chunks) like 'problem', 'fear', 'depression' and 'being stuck' and you don't know what they mean. Here, you can use the NLP meta-model to ask the right questions to chunk down the client's vague words to specific words, thoughts, feelings, and actions (Bandler & Grinder, 1975). Alternatively, we might need to chunk up a client's specific thoughts, feelings, or behaviours to find out their meaning, intention, or category. As hypnotherapists, we often use positive vague terms (high chunks) to induce trance and perform therapy. The client will unconsciously chunk down our vague words to specific positive experiences. We can chunk laterally in the form of metaphors and analogies to open up new ideas and possibilities. In the Spider Phobia session, the client describes her problem in low chunks; she outlines her specific feelings and behaviours when seeing a spider. Brooks chunks up (and thereby reframes) her phobia to the category of learning experiences. He thereby moves it from the negative category of disorders and into the positive category of learnings. This puts her phobia in a row of (positive) learnings, seeding the idea of a learning experience in this session. Later, after transferring the problem from her to the spider, he chunks down to the behaviour and feelings of playing. Then he chunks up again to the values of friendship and care and the identity of a trusted mother. More information about chunking can be found in the NLP literature (O'Connor, 2001).

Mind reading

Mind reading is a linguistic structure in which the hypnotherapist claims to know the client's thoughts or feelings. Milton Erickson was so good at mind reading that many people assumed he had ESP. He always denied this and claimed his knowledge about the client was based on the observation of minimal cues. By reading minimal cues and being artfully vague, he seemed to be able to tell what was on people's minds. Brooks has the same ability, he seems to 'know' what his clients think, feel, believe and need. He garners his information by interpreting a client's words, observing minimal cues, sensing his or her energy, or feeling a spiritual connection. Often, Brooks can't say whether he's used one of these means or a combination of them with a particular client. His mind reading skills are now innate, developed over many years, working with a great number of clients from a range of cultures, ages and lifestyles. Mind reading in Hypnotherapy is a linguistic technique, based on keen observation and the use of artfully vague language and has nothing to do with telepathy or clairvoyance. It can be used to create a yes-set and to pace, ratify or lead the client's experience; it can also increase your perceived authority. Here are some techniques you can use for effective mind reading.

Client's nonverbal language

As a client tells his or her story, he or she will use body language to either support or deny the words that are spoken. Brooks calls this the running commentary of the story. An example of this is a client rubbing his neck while talking about his job. If shown repeatedly, this nonverbal cue could be used at a later stage in the session in the form of mind reading, e.g. "This job is quite a pain in the neck, isn't it?"

Observable emotions

Although each person has a unique way of showing emotions, there are some universal patterns in facial expressions. Paul Ekman has described the typical expression of anger, fear, sadness, disgust, surprise, contempt, and happiness in people all over the world (Ekman, 2003).When a client talks about losing a relative and shows sadness in his or her face, you can say, "Thinking about that makes you feel sad, doesn't it?"

Client's indirect language

Indirect communication is not just used by hypnotherapists. People do it all the time, although they are not usually aware of it. Clients use indirect language, implications, metaphors, analogies, jokes and puns to reveal all kinds of information. Therapists can learn to detect this information and feed it back as a form of mind reading.

Human needs

Although Ericksonian hypnotherapy is very much about individual differences, there are some universal needs that can be addressed in the form of mind reading. Brooks uses a model of 3 basic human needs: 1) the need to know your identity and life purpose; this is also called the need for individuation. 2) the need to belong and to be loved; also known as the need for affiliation. 3) the need for achievement and power. [19] Clients usually reveal their dominant need through their behaviour and words, and you can read their mind by mentioning this. "You really want to find out who you are, don't you?" The client in the Spider Phobia session seems to be driven by the need for affiliation. The problem context she describes at the beginning of the session has mainly to do with home and her family.

Reasonable assumptions

These are statements that can be easily deduced from the client's story or from the very fact that he or she is in therapy. You can say, 'and you are not happy about this, are you?' or 'you have had this problem for some time now'. Again, these things are pretty obvious, but when they are delivered in the right way, they feel very personal to the client.

Wild guess

In addition to the techniques outlined above, you can take a wild guess about the client's thoughts or feelings. The client's response will let you know if you are right, wrong or a little of both. Here, it is important to realise that the client will always respond consciously and unconsciously and that the latter response is more genuine. Oftentimes a wild guess is not as wild as it seems, because unconsciously you may have picked up a lot more about your client than you

[19] Some models have 5 basic human needs; in these, life purpose and power are separate needs.

realise. While the reasonable assumption is based on logic, the wild guess comes from intuition.

With all the mind reading skills above, certain statements might still be experienced by the client as incorrect. This is not a problem as long as you notice it. When the client shows signs of disagreement, you can simply disqualify your remark ("of course I may be totally wrong here...") or offer more possibilities ("or perhaps..."). Sometimes a client may agree with your statement unconsciously by nodding while disagreeing consciously and denying it in words. In Ericksonian hypnotherapy, we usually don't challenge such an incongruity. Rather we respond to both messages, e.g. by also nodding our heads and at the same time admitting that we are wrong. As such, we maintain rapport with both the unconscious and the conscious mind. This way the unconscious can pick up on our statement and use it, although the conscious mind rejects it. Sometimes disagreement from the client can be utilised in a different way. Disagreeing with the therapist can be a way for the client to assert him or herself. In this case, you can repeat your 'wrong' mind-read more strongly to challenge the client to contradict you more firmly. This is the basic principle of Provocative Therapy. In daily life, this principle is used playfully in the form of A: "I bet you can't do this", B: "Yes I can!", A: "No you can't!", B: "Sure I can!!" Although in Ericksonian hypnotherapy the basic principle is not provocation (it is utilisation), it can be used whenever appropriate or effective. Brooks uses mind reading for many purposes: to pace, to normalise, to ratify, to challenge, to provoke, or to predict the client's experience.

Examples from the Spider Phobia session:

> You have a definite strong feeling whenever you fear that a spider.
>
> Yeah, it must be difficult.
>
> You know what the word is, do you not?

Chapter 4: Implication and Presupposition

A special form of indirect communication is the use of implication. An implication is something that is indicated or suggested but not explicitly expressed. Implications are usually not detected by the conscious mind, and therefore they are not criticised or rejected. They are, however, picked up and used by the unconscious. The implication can take many forms, 'linguistic presupposition' is probably the most important one in hypnotherapy. A linguistic presupposition is something that must exist or be true for a sentence to make sense. A simple example is the suggestion "sit down". This suggestion presupposes that the listener is currently standing. Otherwise, the suggestion would not make sense. So, the presupposition of "sit down" is "you are standing". Likewise, the presupposition of the question "when will you do this?" is "you will do this".

An implication is not necessarily a presupposition. A sentence can 'suggest' something to be true but not 'require' (presuppose) it to be true. In linguistics, this type of implication is called an 'implicature', but in this book, we will use the more general term 'implication'. Note that a presupposition or implication is not necessarily verbal; it can also be nonverbal.

In the rest of the book two symbols will be used for presupposition/implication:

> ⊇ means 'presupposes'
>
> ⊃ means 'implies'

Linguistic presuppositions

A linguistic presupposition is a message that is implied with another message. The implied message must be true for the explicit message to make sense. The suggestion,

> Close your eyes

presupposes the listener has his or her eyes open. Presuppositions hold, even if the explicit message is negated. So the suggestion,

Don't close your eyes

also presupposes the listener has his or her eyes open.

All forms of verbal communication, statements, suggestions and questions contain presuppositions. The simple statement "you are here" presupposes a person (you) and a place (here) exist as well as the possibility for 'you to be here'. People are usually unaware of such presuppositions and don't question them. Now, let's look at the following question:

When will you do the dishes?

Presuppositions included in this question are:

There are dishes.

They have not been done yet.

You are able to do the dishes.

You will do the dishes (at a certain time).

The speaker and listener will probably agree on the first three presuppositions without even thinking about it. They might, however, disagree on the fourth one: "You will do the dishes". However, this presupposed (hidden) command is harder to resist than the direct command "Do the dishes". By asking 'when' a certain action will take place, the action itself is presupposed. This form of presupposition is often used to make someone do or admit something so it can be used against a person; for example, a prosecutor asking a suspect "When did you kill the victim?" But it can also be used to benefit someone, for instance a parent asking a child "When will you brush your teeth?" People use linguistic presuppositions all the time, usually without awareness. In fact, any spoken sentence contains multiple presuppositions: about the speaker, the listener, other people or the world. Linguistic presuppositions are used in various forms such as questions, repetitive words, time predicates etc. In this chapter, we will discuss the main presuppositions used by Brooks in his work with clients.

Simple presuppositions

A sentence that refers to a person presupposes that person exists. The statement "My uncle William will visit us tomorrow" presupposes 'my uncle William' exists. The same counts for any object, time, place, state, concept or category that is mentioned in a sentence. "My car has broken down" presupposes 'my car' exists. "I like her a lot" presupposes a specific girl or woman exists. This is fairly obvious for tangible things like people, physical objects, geographical positions, etc. People don't usually question the existence of these things. They might, however, question the existence of intangible things (nominalisations) such as 'hypnosis', 'comfort', 'trance', 'resource', 'goal' or 'solution'. These things do not physically exist in the external world. They cannot be seen or touched. Therefore, they are more likely to be questioned, resisted or denied by the conscious mind. A client might consciously think, "*hypnosis* is nonsense", "I cannot go into *trance*" or "I have no *goal*". If a hypnotherapist uses such words implicitly rather than explicitly, he increases the chance of them bypassing the conscious mind and reaching the unconscious. The unconscious mind can then turn the nominalisation used into a concrete representation, association or action.

Take for example the following sentences which pre-suppose certain nominalisations exist.

I don't know yet how we will find a <u>solution</u>

- Presupposition: there is a solution.

Do you know what <u>your unconscious mind</u> can do for you?

- Presupposition 1: the unconscious mind exists
- Presupposition 2: you have an unconscious mind.

The <u>secret of hypnosis</u> is that things happen all by themselves.

- Presupposition 1: a secret exists
- Presupposition 2: hypnosis exists
- Presupposition 3: hypnosis holds a secret

The idea is that every 'thing' that is mentioned is assumed to exist and will somehow be represented by the listener. How vivid the representation will be, depends on many things. To begin with, the listener needs to know the word. If you read or hear the word 'gezelligheid', you will probably not have any clear representation of it (unless you understand Dutch). When you know a word, you will automatically search for reference experiences (associations). Someone who has never experienced 'hypnotherapy' may have a vague notion of it, while someone who associates it with stage hypnosis might have an entirely false representation.

It is not just the word itself which determines its representation. The way it is delivered is equally important. You could say, "I wonder how hypnosis can help you resolve this issue" in a flat, monotonous voice with a straight face, or you could say it in a melodious voice, stressing the word **hypnosis** while smiling. The client's representation of the word 'hypnosis' may be markedly different depending on which you use. Brooks talks of "communicating emphatically" in respect of this. Think of how great speakers can enchant entire crowds with their use of language and their style of delivery.

A client's inner representation of a certain word can take his or her attention away from the outer world and create a slight trance, even if it is only for a moment. Experienced hypnotists can put people into deep trances simply using a series of nominalisations in an emphatic or engaging way.

Nominalisations are an important area in Ericksonian hypnotherapy. They are vague because they are ideas, concepts, generalisations etc. They are implicative because it is implied they really do exist. Because it is presupposed that they exist, the client will find an inner representation of them.

Questions

Questions always contain presuppositions, things that must be true in order for the question to make sense. Even a one-word question like "How?" presupposes that there is 'something' that happened or will happen and that there is a certain 'way' for it to happen. Typical questions asked in hypnotherapy are those that start with 'who', 'when', 'where', 'what' or 'how'. They often have a twofold intention: gathering information and delivering a message (in the form of a presupposition). The client will usually respond consciously to the information part and will unconsciously pick up on the presupposition. For example:

> Who do you think can support you in this process?
>
> > Presupposition: someone can support you.
>
> When will you go into trance?
>
> > Presupposition: you will go into trance at some point in time.
>
> Where will you find comfort?

Presupposition: you will find comfort at a certain place or from a certain person.

What can we do to make this better?

Presupposition: we can do something to make this better.

How did you manage to get this far?

Presupposition: you managed to get this far in a certain way.

Examples from the Spider Phobia session:

What would you like her to become? ⊇ you'd like her to become something

What comes to mind? ⊇ something comes to mind

How did you feel at that moment? ⊇ you felt something at that moment

How are we gonna free the spider? ⊇ we are going to free the spider in a certain way

Who could she become? ⊇ she can become someone

Sometimes, clients will (consciously) answer these questions by saying "I don't know". The nice thing about Ericksonian hypnotherapy is that you can be pleased with this answer. The conscious mind says, "I don't know" whereas the unconscious can pick up the presupposition and use it. Brooks typically smiles when a client says he or she doesn't know and responds with the suggestion:

"You really don't know, do you?"

It is a gentle way of pacing the client's experience and also downplaying his or her conscious mind. The above questions are direct questions. They can easily be turned into embedded questions with the same presuppositions. This is, so to speak, a way of wrapping up or hiding your message even more.

I wonder, who can support you in this process.
You can be curious, about when you will go into trance.
You may not know yet, where you will find comfort.
I don't know, what we can do to make this better.
I ask myself, how you managed to get this far.

All of the above questions, direct and embedded, are open questions, i.e. they allow for any answer within a certain frame. Certain closed questions hold presuppositions as well, e.g. negatively stated questions. Some examples are:

> Don't you want to experience a new sense of awareness?
>
> > Presupposition: I think you want to experience a new sense of awareness.
>
> Wouldn't you like to let go of those limiting ideas?
>
> > Presupposition: I think you would like to let go of those limiting ideas.

Note that the positively stated version of such a question (Do you want to...) does not hold this presupposition.

Examples from the Spider Phobia session:

> Don't you want to help that little thing? ⊇ I think you want to help that little thing
>
> Don't they always tell you something? ⊇ I think they always tell you something

Factive verbs

Factive verbs are verbs that presuppose the truth or existence of something. They are verbs like 'to know', 'to realise', 'to be aware', 'to remember', 'to discover', 'to notice' and 'to regret'. In hypnotherapy, they are used to presuppose certain statements or suggestions. Some examples are:

> Are you aware, that trance is happening?
>
> > Presupposition: trance is happening.
>
> You may not realise, changes have started to occur.
>
> > Presupposition: changes have started to occur.
>
> Now I know, your unconscious mind can do unbelievable things.
>
> > Presupposition: your unconscious mind can do unbelievable things.
>
> Just notice how things are improving step by step.
>
> > Presupposition: things are improving step by step.

Strictly speaking, factive verbs can only be used with statements or questions, not with commands (suggestions). In hypnotherapy, however, statements often act as suggestions. The statement "your unconscious mind can do unbelievable things" is actually a suggestion for the client's unconscious mind to "do unbelievable things". Factive verbs can refer to the client (you) or the therapist (I). Conscious attention is directed towards awareness of the issue and away from the issue itself.

Examples from the Spider Phobia session:

> You can <u>be aware</u> of the feelings in your arms ⊇ you have feelings in your arms
>
> I <u>know</u> you can write with a laser ⊇ you can write with a laser
>
> She's gonna <u>discover</u> she can change into anything ⊇ she can change into anything
>
> You <u>didn't know</u> that you can find a bunch of wonderful friends ⊇ you can find a bunch of wonderful friends
>
> You <u>know</u> you are going to feel more relaxed ⊇ you are going to feel more relaxed

Relative clauses

A relative clause is a dependent clause that starts with a relative pronoun like 'that', 'who', 'which' or 'what'. It qualifies a noun (or noun phrase) presupposing that noun to exist.

> The *trance* <u>that</u> you were in, was rather deep.
>
> > Presupposition: you were in a trance.
>
> The *answer* <u>which</u> will come up, might surprise you.
>
> > Presupposition: an answer will come up.
>
> The *person* <u>who</u> likes you, is out there somewhere.
>
> > Presupposition: a person likes you.
>
> The *deep state of trance* <u>that</u> you were in proves you are a good hypnotic subject.
>
> > Presupposition: you were in a deep state of trance.

The pronoun 'that' can be omitted if the noun it qualifies is the grammatical object of the sentence. The presupposition is the same.

The *trance* that you were in, was rather deep.

The *trance* you were in, was rather deep.

Examples from the Spider Phobia session:

A woman who had a daddy longlegs phobia ⊇ a woman had a daddy longlegs phobia[20]

Changes that have happened ⊇ changes have happened

Noun clause

A noun clause is a clause that functions as a noun in a sentence. It can be the subject or object of the sentence. Some examples of the former are:

That you have managed to get this far is amazing. [21]

Presupposition: you have managed to get this far.

What happens now will change your life forever.

Presupposition: something happens now.

Examples of the latter are:

You can look at what you have achieved.

Presupposition: you have achieved something.

You will find out that you are worthwhile.

Presupposition: you are worthwhile.

Sometimes a noun clause is reduced to a gerund phrase. Depending on the rest of the sentence and the context, a fact or a possibility is presupposed.

Going into trance was easy after all, wasn't it? [22]

Presupposition: you went into trance. (fact)

---

[20] The more important implication here is: I have helped other people with a similar phobia.

[21] An alternative would be: "It is amazing that you have managed to get this far."

[22] A reduction of "It was easy for you to go into trance after all, wasn't it?"

I recommend <u>taking this first step</u> soon.

Presupposition: you can take this first step. (possibility)

How do you feel about <u>talking about this experience</u>?

Presupposition: you are —or could be— talking about this experience. (fact or possibility)

Examples from the Spider Phobia session:

Do you like <u>what you see</u>? ⊇ you see something

Thinking about, <u>what you've achieved here</u> ⊇ you have achieved something

Ordinal numerals

Ordinal numerals tell the position of something in a list. They are words like 'first', 'second', 'third'… 'last'. Their occurrence presupposes that there were or will be other instances.

So this will be your <u>first</u> experience of hypnosis?

Presupposition: you will have more experiences of hypnosis.

This is the <u>third</u> time you've said you want to change.

Presupposition: you've said you want to change twice before.

Examples from the Spider Phobia session:

Maybe you want to congratulate her for doing the <u>first</u> step ⊇ she will do more steps

The <u>first</u> thing that it is going to project is a still picture ⊇ more things will project

Words like 'another', 'else', 'each', 'next' and 'final' also belong to the same category of presuppositions:

Please give me <u>another</u> example.

Presupposition: you have already given me at least one example.

What <u>else</u> has helped you to do this?

Presupposition: other things have helped you to do this.

Examples from the spider phobia session:

> So it is <u>another</u> learn-problem ⊇ there are other learn-problems
>
> And I'd like you to learn <u>something else</u> ⊇ you've already learned something
>
> That's the <u>next</u> step ⊇ there have already been one or more steps

Subordinate clauses of time

These are dependent clauses that indicate the moment or time period of a certain state, behaviour or event. They are clauses starting with conjunctions like 'before', 'after', 'as', 'while', 'when', 'during', 'once', 'each time' and 'with each'. In Ericksonian hypnotherapy, subordinate clauses of time are often used to link a present or expected behaviour to a desired one. This linking aspect will be further discussed under dependent suggestions in chapter 5. Here we will focus on the presuppositions that subordinate clauses create. Let's look at some examples:

> <u>Before</u> you go into trance, you can close your eyes.
>
> > Presupposition: you will go into trance.
>
> <u>After</u> you have solved this problem, you can decide what to do.
>
> > Presupposition: you will solve this problem.
>
> <u>As</u> you go deeper, memories might come to mind.
>
> > Presupposition: you are going deeper – or you will go deeper.
>
> You can tell me all about it <u>when</u> you feel comfortable enough.
>
> > Presupposition: you will feel comfortable enough.

Note that subordinate clauses of time can be placed before or after the main clause of the sentence.

Examples from the Spider Phobia session:

> <u>Once</u> you are confident with spiders, you will never ever go back ⊇ you will be confident with spiders
>
> Feel the warmth <u>as</u> your eyelids start to get heavy ⊇ your eyelids are starting to get heavy – or – they will start to get heavy
>
> <u>When</u> it starts to lower, I want you to go deeply relaxed ⊇ it will start to lower

Go into a nice deep comfortable, relaxed state <u>before</u> it touches your arm ⊇ it will touch your arm

Change-of-time verbs

Change-of-time verbs express the status or development of a process in time. These are verbs like 'to begin', 'to start', 'to keep on', 'to continue', 'to stay', 'to stop', 'to proceed', 'to go on' and 'to halt'. These words presuppose a process has not yet started, has started, or has been running for a while. Some suggestions with these presuppositions are:

You can <u>continue</u> going into trance.

Presupposition: you are already going into trance.

Just <u>keep on</u> looking for that clue.

Presupposition: you are already looking for that clue.

Do you really want to <u>stop</u> changing now?

Presupposition: you are changing.

And now, you can <u>begin</u> to reorient yourself back to the room.

Presupposition 1: you are not reorienting yourself yet.

Presupposition 2: you can continue to reorient yourself later.

Note that verbs like 'to begin' or 'to start' presuppose two things: that a process has not yet started and that this process has a certain length and can continue later. In all these examples, conscious attention is drawn to the 'starting', 'continuing' or 'stopping' of the process, rather than the process itself. This gives the unconscious a chance to pick up the presupposition of the sentence and to use it.

Examples from the Spider Phobia session:

It <u>starts</u> to get a little bit heavier ⊇ it will continue to get heavier

Things have already <u>started</u> to change ⊇ things will continue to change

So <u>stay</u> back here and look at her lying on the beach ⊇ you are back here

That image or picture <u>starts</u> to form ⊇ that image or picture will continue to form

<u>Stay</u> on the cloud ⊇ you are on the cloud

Change-of-time adverbs

Like change-of-time verbs, change-of-time adverbs say something about the status or development of a process in time. These are words like 'already', 'still', 'yet' and 'anymore'. They presuppose something about the start, duration or ending of the process. For example:

> Are you still holding on to that tension?
>
> > Presupposition: you have been holding on to that tension for a while.
>
> You know, you don't need that fear anymore.
>
> > Presupposition: you needed that fear before.
>
> You are not in trance yet.
>
> > Presupposition: you will be in trance later.
>
> Things have already started to change.
>
> > Presupposition: things were not expected to start changing so soon.

Apart from 'presupposing' things, sentences with 'change-of-time adverbs' can 'imply' other things. These implications are not required to be true (they are not presuppositions); they are however suggested to be true. Sometimes the 'implications' of a sentence are more important than its 'presuppositions'. Let's consider the first two examples given above:

> Are you still holding on to that tension?
>
> > Presupposition: you have been holding on to that tension for a while.
> >
> > Implication: you can let go of that tension now.
>
> You know, you don't need that fear anymore.
>
> > Presupposition: you needed that fear before.
> >
> > Implication: you can let go of that fear.

Examples from the Spider Phobia session:

> Until they just can't wait anymore ⊇ they have been waiting for a long time

Things have already started to change ⊇ things have started to change earlier than expected

She is still lying there looking at the cloud ⊇ she has been lying there for some time

You know you can still control the laser ⊇ you have been able to control it before

Change-of-place verbs

These are verbs that express a change with respect to a person's or an object's location. They are verbs like 'to come',' to go', 'to enter', 'to leave', 'to arrive' and 'to depart'. Sometimes they are used in the form of phrasal verbs like 'to come back' or 'to go out'. In Ericksonian hypnotherapy, locations can be real or imaginary, physical or metaphorical. For example:

Your conscious mind can go to a comfortable place.

Presupposition: your conscious mind is not there now.

Don't leave that state of trance before everything is integrated.

Presupposition: you are in that state of trance now.

You can come back to the here and now.

Presupposition: you are somewhere else (in a trance) now.

Milton Erickson often used the suggestion of leaving a trance to presuppose the client was in a trance. If the client was not in trance, he or she would immediately go into trance to follow the implication. In this way, the suggestion of 'leaving' trance was actually a way of 'inducing' trance.

Examples from the Spider Phobia session:

Let this cloud come down ⊇ the cloud is up now

Go out and find there some good friends ⊇ you are in here now

You can come back to this room ⊇ you are not in this room now

Repetitive cue words

Repetitive cue words express a certain kind of repetition or addition. They are words and phrases like 'back', 'again', 'also', 'another' and 'as well'.

I wonder how you can be happy again.

Presupposition: you have been happy before.

Now you have this possibility as well.

Presupposition: you already had other possibilities.

Actually, the last example can have two different presuppositions, depending on which word is emphasised:

Now you have **this** possibility as well.

Presupposition: you already had other possibilities.

Now **you** have this possibility as well.

Presupposition: someone else already has this possibility.

When no word or both words are emphasised, the conscious mind may take one or the other presupposition, or it may be confused. The unconscious will recognise both and pick the presupposition that fits best.

Examples from the Spider Phobia session:

It is another learn-problem ⊇ there was at least one previous learn-problem

I would like you to also notice, it starts to get a little bit heavier ⊇ you already noticed something

So she feels okay about it as well ⊇ someone else already feels okay about it[23]

Move it back again over there ⊇ you moved it forward before

Listen to her again, saying those things to him ⊇ you listened to her before

You slowly come back to this room ⊇ you were in this room before

Qualifiers

Qualifiers are words that qualify other words or phrases, in this case the subject of a sentence (Bandler & Grinder, 1975). They are words like 'only', 'even', 'just' and 'except'.

---

23 Here, 'she' is the dissociated picture of the client on the beach and the presupposed 'someone else' is the associated client.

Only *you* know what is best for you.

Presupposition: you know what is best for you.

Even *a highly rational person* can go into trance.

Presupposition: a highly rational person can go into trance.

Just *this insight is* all you needed.

Presupposition: this insight is all you needed.

Nothing can keep you from smoking, except *your willpower.*

Presupposition: your willpower can keep you from smoking.

Examples from the Spider Phobia session:

Just *that part of you* is going to help you $\supseteq$ that part of you is going to help you

Qualifying adjectives

Qualifying adjectives attribute a subjective and gradable quality to a noun. They are words like 'deep', 'high', 'small' and 'close'. In hypnotherapy, the noun qualified by such an adjective is often a nominalisation like 'trance', 'step', 'growth', 'goal' or 'life'. Here are some examples:

You can go into a deep *trance.*

Presupposition: you can go into trance.

You can make a small *step* forward.

Presupposition: you can make a step forward.

Qualifying adjectives have a double function. Firstly, they attribute a quality to the noun that follows. In the example above, 'deep' describes the quality (i.e. depth) attributed to the noun 'trance'. Secondly, they turn the suggested noun into a presupposition. A 'deep trance' presupposes a 'trance'. Conscious attention is drawn to whether, or not, the trance will be deep, and away from the question of whether there will be a trance at all. You can agree to the suggestion and go into a deep trance or disagree and go into a light trance. In both cases, you will go into trance because that is presupposed.

Examples from the Spider Phobia session:

Into a nice deep comfortable *relaxed state* $\supseteq$ into a relaxed state

The warm *sun* can shine now ⊇ the sun can shine now

When you're with a close *friend* ⊇ when you're with a friend

Qualifying adverbs

Adverbs attribute a quality to a verb, adjective or another adverb. They are often words ending with 'ly'. Examples include words like 'slowly', 'highly' and 'nicely', which are derived from the corresponding adjectives 'slow', 'high' and 'nice'. Other adverbs are words like 'very', 'too', 'always', 'well', 'still', 'even' and 'just'. Not only do they qualify the process that follows, but they also presuppose it to occur. Here are some examples:

You can *relax* slowly.

Presupposition: you can relax.

This is a highly *interesting* development.

Presupposition: this is an interesting development.

You can go even *deeper.*

Presupposition: you can go deeper.

Sometimes adverbs take the form of adverbial phrases:

You can *go* all the way into trance.

Presupposition: you can go into trance.

Or adverbial clauses [24]:

You will enjoy life like you have never done before.

Just like qualifying adjectives, qualifying adverbs have a double function. Firstly, they attribute a quality to a verb or adjective. In the first example, 'slowly' is the quality attributed to the verb 'to relax'. Secondly, they turn the suggestion into a presupposition. The suggestion "you can relax slowly" presupposes "you can relax". Conscious attention is drawn to whether the relaxation will occur slowly or quickly, and away from the question of whether it will happen at all. The client can agree to the suggestion and relax slowly or disagree and relax quickly. In both cases, relaxation will take place. Brooks frequently uses the word 'just',

[24] An adverbial clause must contain a subject and a verb whereas an adverbial phrase doesn't.

suggesting ease or simplicity and turning the suggestion that follows into a presupposition.

Examples from the Spider Phobia session:

> You will always be very very confident ⊇ you will always be confident
>
> Let all the muscles just become loose ⊇ let all the muscles become loose
>
> Even deeper relaxed ⊇ deeper relaxed
>
> They really trust each other ⊇ they trust each other
>
> You slowly come back to this room ⊇ you come back to this room
>
> Close your eyes all the way ⊇ close your eyes

Superlative adjectives/adverbs

Superlative adjectives are used to compare nouns (e.g. nominalisations), taking the comparison to the highest degree. Examples include words and phrases like 'best', 'easiest', 'deepest', 'simplest', 'most interesting', 'least common' and 'main'. Mentioning the extreme element of a series or collection presupposes the existence of the other elements. For example, 'the farthest star in the universe' presupposes the existence of nearer stars.

Similar to adjectives, superlative adverbs can be used to compare verbs or adjectives and presuppose the smaller actions or qualities. So, 'the person who runs the fastest' presupposes the existence of other people running.

Further examples:

> The main result of hypnosis is problem resolution.
>
> > Presupposition: hypnosis has other results.
>
> Do you know what the best thing about this is?
>
> > Presupposition: there are other good things about this.
>
> Your most valuable resource is your imagination.
>
> > Presupposition: you have other valuable resources.
>
> I wonder which part of your trauma will heal the quickest.
>
> > Presupposition: other parts of your trauma will heal as well.

Besides the creation of presuppositions, superlative adjectives and adverbs give a certain dramatic effect to a suggestion.

Examples from the Spider Phobia session:

> Just be aware which part of your body feels the warmest ⊇ other parts of your body feel warm to a certain extent
>
> The best gifts are the ones that you don't actually get appreciation for ⊇ there are other gifts

Possessive determiners

Possessive determiners are words that attribute the quality of possession to something. They are words like 'my', 'our', 'your', 'his', 'her' and 'their'. They are followed by a noun, which, in hypnotherapy, is usually a nominalisation. A few examples are:

> Your *ability to visualise* makes you a good receptive subject.
>
> Presupposition: you have the ability to visualise.
>
> My *experience* tells me that your problem is solvable.
>
> Presupposition: I have experience.

The last example implies much more than the indicated presupposition. Note the difference between:

> Your problem is solvable.
>
> My experience tells me that your problem is solvable.

In the first, direct statement, 'I' am talking to 'you'. This means you can dispute or reject what I say. In the second statement, a 'vague instance' (my experience) is talking to 'me'. This is difficult for you to dispute because no one is talking to 'you'. Furthermore, the fact that my experience is telling me something implies that I have extensive experience. Whether this is actually true or not, the implication is there, and this compounds my authority and credibility.

Examples from the Spider Phobia session:

> I would like you to, kind of, collect your *thoughts* ⊇ you have thoughts
>
> In her *dream,* she's gonna discover that she's an image ⊇ she will have a dream
>
> Just take your *time*, take your *time* to come back... ⊇ you have time

Demonstrative determiners

Demonstrative determiners are words that indicate the specific existence of something. Some examples would be words like 'this', 'that', 'these' and 'those'.

> You can go back into that trance now.
>
> > Presupposition: there is a specific trance.
>
> These resources are all available to you.
>
> > Presupposition: specific resources exist.

See also Chapter 3 for more information about articles.

Examples from the Spider Phobia session:

> Think about this problem you've got ⊇ you've got a specific problem
>
> Just that part of you that's going to help you ⊇ you have a specific part
>
> That flutter in your eyelids is an important, integral part of making these changes happen ⊇ there is a specific flutter, and there are specific changes

(Pseudo -) Cleft sentences

Cleft sentences are structures of the form, "it is/was <noun phrase>". A few examples are:

> It is *your tenacity* that will get you through this.
>
> > Presupposition: something will get you through this.
>
> It was *this memory* that you needed.
>
> > Presupposition: you needed something.

With cleft sentences, attention is drawn to the first part of the sentence and away from the second part (the actual suggestion). In the first example above, the client is guided to consciously think about his or her tenacity, while her unconscious picks up on the implication: something will get me through this.

Pseudo-cleft sentences are structures of the form: "<what-clause>...is/was...". A few examples are:

> What you can do is, to lean back and rest.
>
> > Presupposition: you can do *something*.
>
> What I would like you to imagine is, an old tree.

Presupposition: I would like you to imagine *something*.

Pseudo-clefts can also start with 'all' or 'the only/first/next/last thing' instead of a what-clause. Some examples are:

All you need to do is take a first step.

Presupposition: you need to do *something*.

The first thing we should do is to make a plan.

Presupposition: we should do *something*.

Reverse pseudo-cleft sentences [25] are structures of the form "<noun phrase>…is/was what". Some examples are:

A different approach is what will help you resolve this issue.

Presupposition: *something* will help you resolve this issue.

That's what will arise when you let this go.

Presupposition: *something* will arise when you let this go.

Note that all presuppositions created with (pseudo) cleft sentences contain the vague word *something*. Take one of the above examples:

What you can do is, to lean back and rest.

The first part of the sentence:

what you can do is…

presupposes

you can do *something*.

The conscious mind may not pick up the presupposition and wait expectantly for the sentence to be completed. The unconscious will pick up the presupposition, wonder what *something* could mean and will get ready to respond. The second part of the sentence:

...to lean back and rest

specifies what to do. Now the conscious mind is satisfied, and the unconscious can follow the suggestion. So, the trick is to presuppose something vague, and then make it specific. It's very hard for the conscious mind to resist and very

[25] Also called inverted WH-clefts.

easy for the unconscious to follow. Also, you can play a little with analogue marking and use emphasis and a pause:

> What you can **do** is...........

The emphasis on the word '**do**' encourages the client to perform a certain behaviour. The longer the therapist pauses after this part, the more curious the conscious mind will become and the more the unconscious will explore what it 'can do', and therefore might start 'doing' it. Suppose for example that you observe the initial signs of eye closure, then you can include that in your suggestion:

> What you can **do** is........... that's right, close your eyes...and lean back and rest.

Ericksonian hypnotherapy is always about observation/utilisation. When Brooks is working with a client, he will constantly adapt his words to the client's responses. This flexibility with speech is at least as important as the ability to be indirect, implicit and vague.

Examples from the Spider Phobia session:

> <u>What</u> I would like you to do, you know, <u>is</u> you have control over the cloud as well ⊇ I would like you to do something
>
> <u>What</u> I want you to do, <u>is</u> ask her to look at it ⊇ I want you to do something
>
> <u>All</u> it needs <u>is</u> for you to trust it ⊇ it needs something
>
> <u>That's what</u> he's saying as he looks up to you ⊇ he's saying something as he looks up
>
> <u>The next thing</u> for you (to do) <u>is</u> to spend some time ⊇ there is something for you to do

Note that the first sentence is ill-formed, probably intentionally.

Counterfactual conditional clause

A counterfactual conditional clause is a sentence of the form 'if...had/was/would...', suggesting that whatever follows is not true. Some examples are:

If you had never experienced trance before, it would not be so easy.

Presupposition: you have experienced trance before.

Had you not been able to do this, I would have done it for you.

Presupposition: you were able to do this.

Examples from the Spider Phobia session:

If it (the problem) was something that was organic ⊇ it is not organic

Noun-preposition

These are sentences of the form 'The <noun phrase> <preposition> <noun phrase>...is...' with prepositions like 'about' and 'of'. For example:

The wonderful thing about trance is that it happens all by itself.

Presupposition: there is *something wonderful* about trance.

The good side of this is, that you have learned something new.

Presupposition: there is *a good side* of this.

The positive aspect of having gone through this is, that it keeps you alert.

Presupposition: having gone through this has *a positive aspect.*

Note that these examples contain a presupposition and an embedded suggestion. Consider the following example:

The interesting thing about trance is that *it happens all by itself.*

Presupposition: there is something interesting about trance.

Embedded suggestion: *it happens all by itself.*

The word 'it' obviously refers to the word 'trance' and the conscious mind will understand it as such. Nevertheless, 'it' is an unspecified reference and the unconscious can apply it to anything that needs to '*happen all by itself*'.

Examples from the Spider Phobia session:

The good thing about it being learned is that it can be unlearned ⊇ there is something good about it being learned

The wonderful thing about this is that it's all yours ⊇ there is something wonderful about this

Binds and double binds

A special type of linguistic presupposition, often used by Milton Erickson, are binds and double binds. A bind is a question or statement that gives the client an illusion of choice; whatever he or she chooses will lead to the same result. A simple example of a bind is the question: "Do you want coffee or tea?" The presupposition of this question is that the listener wants something to drink. He or she has a choice of what to drink, but the option of taking nothing is not offered. Binds are used in everyday conversation —for example by reporters, salespeople and attorneys— often to manipulate people into admitting or buying something. A car salesman might ask, "Which one do you like more, the Fiat or the Ford?" Whichever you choose, you are on your way to buying a car. Parents often use binds to get their children to do something that needs to be done. They say things like, "Do you want to brush your teeth before or after you put on your pyjamas?" In Ericksonian hypnotherapy, binds are used to lead the client in a therapeutic direction while giving him or her a choice of how to get there. This gives the client a sense of power and the freedom to choose his or her own way of changing. Furthermore, the illusionary choice distracts the conscious mind so that the unconscious can easily pick up and follow the presupposed suggestion. In addition to binds, we use double binds where the client can only choose at the unconscious level. Binds and double binds allow us to circumvent conscious resistance and elegantly lead people in the direction of their own goals.

Binds

When we use a bind, the client is offered a choice that can be made at a conscious level. Whatever he or she chooses, the underlying assumption is accepted.

> Do you want to *go into trance* <u>in this chair or in that chair</u>?

No matter which chair the client chooses, he or she accepts the idea of going into trance.

> Would you prefer *to stop smoking* <u>immediately or gradually over time</u>?

Whichever way the client prefers, he or she is agreeing to the idea of stopping smoking. The choices in these examples are made consciously.

Double bind

With a double bind, the client is offered a choice that he or she can only make at the unconscious level. As Milton Erickson put it:

> "When the patient's conscious mind can discriminate and make a choice between the alternatives, we speak of a bind. When the conscious mind cannot make a choice between the alternatives, we may more properly speak of a double bind because choice is then relegated to responding on another level. This other level sometimes termed a metalevel, can be conceptualised as an unconscious or autonomous mental process." (Erickson & Rossi, 1980)

Some examples are:

Will <u>your right hand or your left hand</u> *start lifting all by itself*?

In order to answer this question, the client can only wait and see which hand will lift. The client will typically say, "I don't know", or say nothing and wait for something to happen. The presupposition of this suggestion is that one of the hands will lift.

Will that tension in your chest <u>increase or decrease</u>?

Again, the client will probably not know what will happen and will wait for an unconscious physical response. The fact that the tension will change is implied. Double binds not only bind the client to the implied suggestion, but they also depotentiate the conscious in favour of the unconscious. Whether something is a bind or a double bind is not always known at the outset. It depends on the client's response. If he or she chooses consciously, it is a bind. If he or she waits for the unconscious to respond, it's a double bind. Nevertheless, some questions are more likely to act as binds whereas others are usually experienced as double binds. Binds are often used at the beginning of a session when the conversation is mainly at the conscious level. A couple of simple binds that I (JvB) use at the beginning of a session are "Do you want coffee, tea or water?" and "You can hang your coat up here or put it down there". These are innocuous choices that the client can easily make. Later in the session, I'll use more challenging binds and, whenever I use hypnosis, double binds.

Note that double binds can be presented in the form of a direct or embedded question, or a direct or embedded statement. [26]

> Direct question: Will your left hand or your right hand get numb?
>
> Embedded question: I wonder whether your left hand or your right hand will get numb.
>
> Direct statement: Your left hand or your right hand will get numb.
>
> Embedded statement: It will be interesting to find out whether your left hand or your right hand will get numb.

Examples from the Spider Phobia session:

> *Some cloud up there*, and it is to your left or to your right?

Time (double) bind

With a time bind suggestion, the illusionary choice refers to the time that a suggested response will occur.

> Would you like to *talk about this* now or later?

Here, the client can make a conscious choice about 'when' he or she wants to talk about a certain issue. The fact that it will be talked about it is implied.

> I wonder whether *the experience of trance will occur* this session or next time.

The question is not whether trance will happen or not; it's a matter of when. Since the client cannot go into trance consciously, she will typically wonder and wait for trance to happen. The words 'occur' and 'happen' encourage the unconscious mind to respond rather than the conscious mind, and make this suggestion a double-bind.

Examples from the Spider Phobia session:

> And you can wonder whether you *go all the way down into a nice deep comfortable, relaxed state* before it touches your arm.

Note that in this example the only time reference for something to happen is 'before it touches your arm'. The alternative (after it touches your arm) is not mentioned; it is implied.

---

[26] Both questions and statements can act like suggestions.

Verbal implications

So far, we have discussed various types of presuppositions: things that must be true for the suggestion to make sense. However, not all implications are presuppositions. A sentence can imply various things without requiring (presupposing) them to be true. The listener unconsciously just assumes these things to be true, based on expectations, ideas and beliefs about himself, other people or the world. Consider the following request:

> Please give me a glass of water.
>
> > Presupposition: water and a glass are available.
> >
> > Implication: the speaker will drink the water.

The availability of water and a glass is a prerequisite (presupposed) for this request to make sense. The assumption that the water will be drunk is not necessarily correct. It might be used for other purposes or not at all. Linguistically, the sentence "Please give me a glass of water" makes sense, even if you don't drink it. Presuppositions are well defined, and they are determined by the words themselves. The sender and receiver of a message usually agree on presuppositions, although they might not be aware of them. Implications depend on context, available information, expectations and beliefs. So, sender and receiver might disagree on the implications. Suppose your partner asks you:

> Can you water the plants today?
>
> > Presupposition: there are plants, and you are able to water them.
> >
> > Implication: the plants need water.

You will probably agree on the presuppositions. You don't need to think about them. You might, however, disagree on whether the plants need water today. That is your partner's assumption. She might ratify it with her choice of words, voice tone or body language. She might say for example, "Can you water the plants today, please?" while pointing at the dry soil of a particular plant. Still, she doesn't say "The plants need water". That is implied, albeit more strongly now. The implication in this example is obvious, but that is not always the case. Many questions, statements or suggestions have implications that are very subtle and not so easy to recognise. Let's have a look at some specific forms of implications.

Time adverbs

Time adverbs are adverbs that refer to the time or frequency of an event, state or action. As described in Chapter 2, they can be used to create embedded suggestions. When used with statements rather than suggestions, time adverbs can also create an implication. The more the time adverb is emphasised, the stronger the implication. For example:

> I know it looks bad now.
>
> > Implication: it will look better later.
>
> You were confused then.
>
> > Implication: you are not confused now.
>
> Sometimes you don't know what to do.
>
> > Implication: other times you do know what to do.

Statements like these are often used to acknowledge or normalise the client's negative experience. Slightly emphasising the time adverb of the statement implies its opposite and indirectly leads the client to a positive experience.

Note that time adverbs like 'now' and 'later' create implications (things 'assumed' to be true) whereas change-of-time adverbs like 'still' and 'yet' create presuppositions (things 'required' to be true).

> You are not happy now.
>
> > Implication: you will be happy later. [27]
>
> You are not happy yet.
>
> > Presupposition: you will be happy later.

Examples from the Spider Phobia session:

> And your mum couldn't help it back then.

Verb tenses

Here the tense of a verb is used to imply something is in the 'past', 'present' or 'future'. Some examples are:

> What was the problem?

---

[27] Or "you were happy before", depending on context.

Implication: it is not a problem anymore.

Someday you will be old and grey.

Implication: you are not old and grey now.

Brooks often uses a combination of time adverbs and verb tenses, for example:

Look at the problem you had, back then.

Not only will he emphasise these words but also direct his voice to a location behind the client to further strengthen the suggestion that the problem is in the past (behind you). Directing your voice at different locations for different times is a form of analogue marking.

Examples from the Spider Phobia session:

And what else would you have liked to have heard in the past, when you had your problem before, in the past?

Notice how you used to feel before, if you had thought of a spider.

Implicative verbs

All verbs imply something, e.g. the existence of the action they describe. Some verbs, however, have very interesting or useful implications. Some examples might be:

You have managed to make it better.

Implication: making it better wasn't easy.

You can try to open your eyes.

Implication: opening your eyes will be difficult/impossible.

You have dared to confront him.

Implication: confronting him was challenging/frightening for you.

Wonderful things can happen.

Implication: you don't have to do anything, they happen automatically.

I congratulate you for making this decision.

Implication: making this decision is a positive event/result.

You can learn to express your feelings.

Implication: expressing your feelings is interesting or valuable.

The use of some verbs is a bit tricky because they also have certain presuppositions. Take the following sentence:

You can learn to play the piano.

Presupposition: you cannot play the piano now.

Implication: playing the piano is interesting or valuable.

If the listener cannot play the piano, the presupposition matches the truth, and the implication can motivate him or her to start playing. If, however, the listener can play or thinks he or she can play, he or she might feel insulted or belittled, even without consciously recognising the presupposition. Brooks uses the word 'learn' several times during the Spider Phobia session, e.g. "…learn to leave that problem in the past". Here it is obvious that, so far, the client has not been able to leave her problem in the past, so the presupposition of this suggestion matches her experience, and the implication can help her solve the problem.

Examples from the Spider Phobia session:

Learn to leave that problem in the past ⊃ leaving the problem in the past is valuable.

What you manage to do for yourself ⊃ what you do for yourself is an achievement.

Simply by us talking, things have started to happen ⊃ things happen automatically.

Utilising beliefs

Unlike presuppositions, implications depend on context and beliefs. As well as general beliefs shared by people of the same culture, people have their own individual beliefs, assumptions, expectations and meanings. Once you know your client's beliefs, you can use them for implication. To a Christian client who suppresses his anger and has difficulty being assertive, you could say:

Even Jesus became angry at the money-changers and threw them out of the temple.

This statement holds the implication that anger and acting assertively is acceptable. Obviously, this implication is only valid for someone who assumes that Jesus existed and that he was good. Note the meaning of the word 'even'. It implies Jesus was someone special, not expected to be angry or aggressive. The fact that he was angry 'anyway', strengthens the idea that expressing anger is acceptable.

Nonverbal implications

Any context, situation, event or behaviour implies certain things exist or are true. The context of a hospital implies the existence of doctors, nurses, beds and medical equipment. It also implies the existence and importance of medical investigation and treatment. A church service is an event that implies the presence of a priest and the existence of religion and God. The behaviour of driving a car implies the driver possesses a driver's licence and has a certain destination. Although all of these implications are not necessarily true, they are assumed to be true by the observer or listener. A hypnotherapy practice implies the presence of a hypnotherapist and the possibility of a hypnotherapy session. As a hypnotherapist, you can use this principle to choose or create a context with powerful implications. Some examples are:

> A plaque on your door saying "Certified Hypnotherapist".
>
> > Implication: You are an expert in hypnosis.
>
> A full —or seemingly full— work schedule.
>
> > Implication: You are busy, which implies you are good.

The very fact that you're a 'hypnotherapist' implies that 'hypnosis' will be used and that the effect will be 'therapeutic'. Any aspect of your practice context (office, website, flyers, certificates etc.) can be used to strengthen this idea. Brooks is a very successful hypnotherapist. Many clients know this beforehand and assume that having therapy with him will help them. Brooks utilises this belief and often compounds it by referring to previous successful treatments. The setting for the demonstration described in this book is a stage with an audience and a camera. This implies that the client's process will be interesting and valuable to others. Brooks verbally reinforces this nonverbal implication, by thanking the client for coming. Of course, implications only work if they are picked up and accepted by the client's unconscious mind. If the client has never heard of hypnotherapy, the term will not imply anything.

The context used for implication can be real or imaginary. A visualised context has the same implications as a real one. In the Spider Phobia session, Brooks sets up the visualised context of a beach with clouds in the sky. The context of a beach on a summer day implies warmth, open space, fun, relaxation etc. Clouds have the implication of temporariness, movement and vagueness. At the end of the session, Brooks leads the client through a game with a spider, implying playfulness, joy and freedom. An imaginary context may include symbols and archetypes with their own implications. The symbol of a 'wall' implies separation or captivity whereas a 'key' implies access or solution. The archetype 'mother' implies care and protection whereas the archetype 'lion' implies power and danger. Brooks uses the symbol of a 'ring' at the beginning of the session, which may imply connection, loyalty or trust for the client. Later, he uses the archetype of the (close) 'friend', which implies kindness, trust, etc.

Nonverbal implication also refers to the para-verbal aspects of speech like voice tone, pitch, volume, tempo, emphasis and pauses. Pausing in the middle of a sentence implies that something important is to come; it builds up expectation.

> I wonder if you can……allow that feeling to get stronger.

A pause after a question or suggestion implies an answer or response is expected. Milton Erickson often mentioned the power of 'waiting expectantly', meaning pausing with an open and curious expression and posture.

The para-verbal implication can also be used to strengthen or change a verbal implication. Let's look at another example: "You were powerless then". The greater the emphasis on the word **then**, the stronger the implication of "You are not powerless now". Emphasising other words, however, changes the implication of the sentence.

> You were powerless **then**.
>
> > Implication: you are not powerless now.
>
> You were **powerless** then.
>
> > Implication: it was not your fault.
>
> **You** were powerless then.
>
> > Implication: someone else had the power.

Even a one-word question like "Why?" or "Really?" can express surprise, curiosity, doubt or disbelief, depending on the way it is pronounced. Any form of analogue marking, voice tone, volume, pitch, stretching a word, gesture or facial expression can be used to control the implications in a sentence. Brooks constantly uses verbal and nonverbal forms of implication. He uses them to imply general things like change, growth, healing, success and happiness or more specific things relevant to the client's problem or symptom. He considers implied messages to be more effective than explicit ones.

Implication and relevance

Although every utterance contains presuppositions and implications, not every one of them is therapeutically relevant. If your client has just entered your office and you say, "Please, sit down", this implies the client is standing. However, this is obvious and usually not something you want to point out. Your intended message is the explicit "sit down", not the implied "you are standing". If, however, during the therapeutic process you say, "you just took the first step", your intended message might be the implied one: "there will be more steps". Whether or not an implication is relevant also depends on the client's knowledge and expectations. If a client knows at the outset that there will be several steps —and accepts this— the statement "you just took the first step" is a mere conclusion and the implication "there will be more steps" is not so relevant.

Chapter 5: Splitting and Linking

Since ancient times, human beings have had a desire to understand and make sense of the world, life and themselves. Understanding any object, organism or process involves knowing its basic elements and the relationship between those elements. A drop of water can be seen as one fluid and transparent thing or as trillions of H2O molecules held together by electrical forces. The human body can be seen as a whole, or as a collection of organic cells. Both perspectives have their advantages and disadvantages. Seeing the whole of something allows you to simply use or enjoy it. Seeing the components allows you to understand, change or recreate it.

Using the basic principle of splitting the whole and (re)linking components, humans have influenced nature, created cultures and developed technology. Scientists and technicians have created a wealth of products including chemicals, materials, objects, machines and computers. Biologists have discovered cells as the building blocks of living organisms, DNA molecules as the carriers of all genetic material and thousands of biochemical substances controlling our physiology. Medical scientists and doctors use splitting and linking at the level of molecules, cells, DNA, and organs to prevent infection, heal wounds and cure diseases.[28]

In the physical world, the components of a system are concrete and the links between them real. The human mind, however, also creates conceptual splits and links. We make all kinds of distinctions which do not exist in the outside world but are created in our minds. We split time into past, present and future, the world into different countries and cities, people into friends and enemies and ourselves into body and mind. None of these splits is concrete or even real, but we experience them as real by naming and visualising them and believing them to be true.

As well as making splits, we connect (link) all kinds of things that are not necessarily related. We link events to consequences (e.g. this failure 'will get me' fired), perceptions to feelings (e.g. seeing him struggle 'makes me' sad) or behaviours to meanings (this relapse 'means' I am weak). Often these links act like self-fulfilling prophecies; they become real because we think and behave as if they are. Conceptual splits and links can support or limit our health, success or happiness. For example, someone who assumes a strict separation (split) of body and mind might find it difficult to relate headaches to stress; he or she will

[28] Whether our influence on —and control of— nature is a good thing is, of course, a matter of opinion.

use medication rather than trying relaxation exercises or considering a change of lifestyle. Someone who attributes (links) his depression to his partner's behaviour will not be motivated to change. Depending on culture, life experiences, education and profession, people create all kinds of conceptual splits and links, some supporting, others limiting their lives. Part of our job as hypnotherapists is to remove limiting links and strengthen or create supporting ones. The question, however, is what are the basic components of human experience and how are they linked together? Most psychotherapeutic approaches in the western world [29] agree that the following elements influence experience:

- The body with its organs, cells, genes, nervous system, hormone system and sensory organs.
- Sensory perception of the environment through images, sound, taste, smell and touch.
- Behaviour: actions, movements, gestures, facial expressions etc.
- Thoughts: internal images or self-talk
- Physical feelings: tactile, visceral, or proprioceptive sensations
- Emotions: basic (like fear, anger, sadness, happiness) and social (like guilt and shame)
- Sensory representation of past experiences (memories)
- Sensory representation of future experiences (plans, dreams, fantasies)
- Meanings, interpretations, conclusions, expectations: ideas about perceived objects, events, actions, feelings etc.
- Beliefs, norms, and values: long-term stable ideas about self, others and the world.
- Social relationships: representations of family, friends and colleagues.

Therapeutic orientations, however, differ widely in their assumptions of the relation between these components. Each discipline has its own idea about the nature of a psychological problem, its cause and its solution. Psychoanalytic therapists tend to see problems as unconscious conflicts, rooted in past trauma

[29] Eastern approaches also distinguish the chakras and meridians, while Shamanists view the soul as a part of human experience.

that can be resolved through insight. Behavioural therapists consider problematic behaviour to be the result of classical and operant conditioning and use desensitisation and the development of behavioural skills. Cognitive therapists consider irrational beliefs to be the cause of psychological suffering and view the awareness and conscious change of those beliefs as the solution. Humanistic therapists consider that the lack of opportunity to actualise potential and talent is the cause of problems; they see creating those opportunities as the solution.

Milton Erickson believed that problems arise from limited conscious ideas and patterns; he advocated evoking unconscious resources as the solution. Other than this general principle, he had no predefined theory about psychological problems, causes and solutions. Instead, he emphasised the importance of discovering the client's unique associational network (splits and links) and utilising this for trance and therapeutic change. Limiting splits/links can be challenged, changed, removed or utilised as part of a solution. Supporting splits/links are activated, strengthened, or created. As such, Ericksonian hypnotherapy can involve any therapeutic pathway such as trauma resolution, desensitisation, pattern interruption, behavioural change, skill development, belief change, social reconstruction, the creation of opportunity or spiritual growth, as long as it resonates with the client's resources, beliefs and needs. Many clients experience a limiting link between a perception —e.g. an image or a sound— and a negative feeling. In this book, we study a session with a woman who has a spider phobia. Her limiting link is between the image (externally or internally) of a spider and an intense feeling of fear. Her therapy includes removing that link and replacing it with a supporting one; seeing a spider evokes a state of connection and care. Apart from a client's personal associational network, Erickson used various splits and links that are universal parts of the human experience. These include:

- Consciousness: conscious/unconscious
- Time: past/present/future, old/young, long/short
- Space: here/there, left/right, up/down

Bill O'Hanlon has described how Erickson used splitting and linking to induce trance or practise therapy, identifying his use of time, space, body parts, voice tone and various other distinctions (O'Hanlon, 1987). The splitting of the conscious and the unconscious is a central element of trance induction and therapy. On trance termination, the conscious and unconscious are re-associated, usually in a better way than before.

As Milton Erickson wrote:

> The induction and maintenance of a trance serve to provide a special psychological state in which the patient can re-associate and reorganise his inner psychological complexities and utilise his own capacities in a manner concordant with his own experiential life (Erickson & Rossi, 1979).

Development of splits and links

A person's associational network develops throughout the course of his or her life. A new-born baby has only a limited set of sensory responses —for example, an aversion to bitter substances— and motor reflexes as, for example, the suck and grasp reflex. These are instinctive stimulus-response links. From the moment of birth, a lifelong process of learning begins. A large network of links starts to develop between all kinds of stimuli and learned responses (classical conditioning). Seeing mother's face can be linked to a sense of comfort and the behaviour of smiling. Hearing a dog's loud barking could be linked to a feeling of fear. Other links arise between certain behaviours and positive or negative consequences (operant conditioning). A child saying his or her first words can be rewarded (and linked) with smiles and encouraging words. Throwing food may be punished (and linked) with a harsh voice or an angry face. As time goes by many links will fade and die as particular stimuli or consequences disappear or are overtaken by stronger links. Others become a, more or less, permanent part of the child's associational network. Any split or link in this network can be supporting or limiting, depending on how it affects behaviour, thinking and feeling. A spider phobia, for example, is a conditioned link between the image of a spider and the feeling of intense fear, often accompanied by the behaviour of avoidance. For most people, this is a very limiting link.

After his or her first few years, the learning of a child becomes more cognitive and symbolic, especially when language develops. The child not only learns about the actual consequences of his or her behaviour from experience (holding your finger in a candle flame hurts) but also about possible consequences from verbal messages ("If you do your homework now, you can watch television later"). Besides possible consequences, the child's behaviour becomes more and more connected to meaning. Good grades in school might get the meaning "I am a good boy". Fighting with other children could mean "there is something wrong with me". Not just behaviours but also emotions get meaning. Crying for a boy might mean "being weak" whereas for a girl it could mean "being sensitive". Even meanings get meaning. Clients with a fear of failure have often developed the link: 'making a mistake' means 'I failed' which in turn means 'I am a failure'. Meanings do not exist in the external world; they exist only in people's minds. And although they are neither true nor untrue, people experience them as an existing truth. All in all, a vast network of associations develops in a person's mind: links between events, behaviours, emotions, consequences and meanings. Some are automatic and unconscious and are stored in the implicit memory; others are more cognitive and are stored in the explicit memory. In NLP, this individual network of links is called the 'model of the world': the model each person creates of him or herself and the world. Although people have very different models of the world, most people experience their own model as the truth, as the way it is. They experience their responses, emotions, and meanings as normal and right. As far as the physical world is concerned, there is an observable truth. The chair you are sitting on exists, as does the book you are reading. People usually agree on the existence of observable things[30]. In the mental, emotional and spiritual world, however, there is no observable truth. There is only interpretation, association, assumption, conclusion, expectation, meaning and belief: all things we construct in our minds. Most people, it seems, need a certain truth. Our conditioned responses and beliefs tell us, in any given situation, what is true, and therefore what to do, how to feel and what to say. But some responses or beliefs are so limiting that we need to break them in order to live a happy or successful life.

As well as making countless links, a child learns to make distinctions, i.e. he or she learns to split the world into parts. For a new-born baby, the world and everyone in it are probably one, and there is only 'now'. Soon, the infant discovers itself to be separate from its mother and that its right hand is its own but different from the left. He or she learns to distinguish various objects, materials and substances: some solid, some fluid, some moving and others still. Later, the child learns how living things are divided into plants, animals and people and, in turn, people are categorised as boys and girls, adults and children, friends and enemies etc. [31] The child learns about conceptual splits of time (past, present, future), place (here, there, far away), possession (my things, your things), language (letters, words, sentences, stories) and judgment (good/bad, right/wrong, legal/illegal). As with links, the splits in your associational network can be limiting or supporting. A strong separation between past and future can help you to leave a bad experience behind, but it can also prevent you from learning from it and integrating it into your present and future.

---

[30] Except for people with hallucinations, either from psychological disorder or hypnotic trance.

[31] This division into groups is a process of both splitting and linking.

Removing limiting links

Hypnotherapy often involves the weakening or removal of limiting links. It can be used to influence conditioned responses and cognitive beliefs. Conditioned responses are treated with hypnotic desensitisation, dissociation and indirect suggestions. Limiting beliefs can be changed in various ways. In the field of NLP, Robert Dilts has developed NLP interventions (Dilts R. B., 1990) (Dilts, Hallbom, & Smith, 1990) as well as conversational techniques (Dilts R. B., 1999) to change limiting beliefs. Milton Erickson often changed a limiting belief by suggesting the opposite or by creating a dramatic experience[32] that proved the opposite. Brooks has a background in both Ericksonian hypnotherapy and NLP and uses all of these methods to work with beliefs. Conversationally, he might start by casting some doubt on the client's expressed belief. In the Spider Phobia session, he simply repeats the question "Really?" several times to challenge the belief "my phobia is an inherited problem".[33] He uses the trance experience of dissociation as a demonstration of the client being in control; the opposite of her usual experience with spiders. He has her visualise helping a scared spider, an imaginary experience that counteracts her belief that she is the scared one who needs help. Throughout the session he gives her suggestions of 'doing' okay and 'being' okay, challenging any possible beliefs of the opposite. At the end of the session, he uses arm catalepsy as a metaphor for the client's strength, counteracting her belief in her own helplessness. Many of her obvious beliefs and possible beliefs are dealt with without them even being mentioned. In Ericksonian hypnotherapy, clients may or may not become aware of a belief change after it has happened. At the end of the session, Brooks asks the client, "How did you do that?" referring to the reduction of her fear from 10 to 0. She shrugs her shoulders and says "I don't know". This means she doesn't know consciously, which is fine. Brooks didn't ask this question to get a conscious answer. He asks it specifically to imply that 'she' did it and to ratify that belief. The client is surprised that her conditioned response to the thought of a spider has disappeared. She cannot fully believe it yet. Brooks gives her the task of finding spiders in the building as a final step of solidifying and ratifying the change that has happened. She finds out that her conditioned response to seeing a real spider has disappeared as well. These experiences both confirm and strengthen her beliefs about being in control and solving the problem herself. During the session, Brooks planted many seeds for self-confidence and self-esteem which she might become aware of in time. Or, she might just enjoy their

---

[32] In the form of a trance experience or a task to be performed in daily life.

[33] Actually, he asks this question indirectly as part of a story about a different client.

effect in the form of positive feelings and useful behaviour. In the next paragraph, I describe the various linguistic patterns Brooks uses to create supporting links.

Creating constructive links

Ericksonian hypnotherapy offers many ways of creating or building new links, associations and beliefs. Such links can be set up for trance induction, for therapeutic change or for both. A common technique is to suggest a link between a current state and a desired state.

> Sitting in that chair can LEAD TO a sense of comfort.

Sitting in the chair is an observable fact so when mentioned the client can easily agree creating a yes-set. A sense of comfort is now more easily accepted and experienced, because of the yes-set, along with the idea that it results from sitting in the chair. The link can be temporary, helping the client to experience comfort in the session, or it can become permanent by generalisation (sitting in a chair leads to comfort). If necessary, this generalisation can be enhanced in the form of a posthypnotic suggestion:

> Any time you sit in a chair like that, you will *feel comfortable.*

or more indirectly:

> I wonder if that *sense of comfort* will come up before or after you sit down in your office chair, and whether this new experience will start on a Monday, Tuesday, Wednesday, or Thursday.

Let's have a look at the various language patterns Brooks uses to create links.

Adjunctive suggestions

Adjunctive suggestions[34] link one state or idea to another state or idea, using words like 'and', 'but', 'yet', 'even', 'if' or 'still'.

Connecting related states or processes

The simplest and most common form of adjunctive suggestions connects a current state or idea to a desired one with the word 'and'.

---

[34] They are also referred to as compound suggestions (Erickson & Rossi, 1981).

Some examples are:

> You are sitting here AND you can feel comfortable.
>
> > The current state (sitting here) is an observable fact.
>
> Your hands are on your lap AND you can notice how they feel.
>
> > Again, the current state is an observable fact.
>
> You can hear the sound of my voice AND simply start to relax.
>
> > The current state is not an observable fact, but very likely to be true.
>
> I know you want to change your behaviour AND now you can learn how to do that.
>
> > The current state is not an observable fact, but can be a result of the pre-talk or a reasonable assumption when the client has come to therapy voluntarily.
>
> Thoughts go through your mind AND they can gradually fade away.
>
> > The current state is not an observable fact, but a reasonable assumption when the client is not in a deep trance.

Whether the current state is an observable fact, shared information or a reasonable assumption doesn't matter. What counts is that the client says YES to it. In that case, a yes-set is established and the client is likely to accept what follows. The link between the two states is not necessarily logical or factual. It is created based on the truism of the current state, the word AND, plus the suggestion of the desired state. In the above examples, the current state precedes the desired state. Sometimes, however, the order is reversed. In that case, the current state has a slightly different function. It reinforces the suggested desired state after it has been delivered. (Erickson, Rossi, & Rossi, 1976)

> You can feel comfortable AND you can hear my voice.

Apart from being 'current' or 'desired', states can be 'observable' or 'non-observable'. Observable states can be observed from the outside. They are behaviours, postures, movements, gestures, facial expressions and physical responses. Some examples are sitting, standing, moving, fidgeting, nodding, breathing, blinking and sighing. They are things other people can see or hear.

Non-observable states cannot be directly observed from the outside. Examples are physical feelings, emotions, thoughts and mental images. These states are internal to the client. They can, however, become observable by the minimal cues they produce. Relaxation can result in the flattening of facial muscles or stillness of the body, emotions show themselves in facial expressions (Ekman, 2003) while thoughts can be revealed by eye movements (O'Connor, 2001). Conflict resolution and relaxation often trigger audible, visceral sounds. As soon as a desired state has become a current state, it can be linked to a new desired state. A therapist adopting Ericksonian hypnotherapy needs to be skilled in observing minimal cues in order to follow this process of developing states of trance. Brooks often uses serial suggestions (series of adjunctive suggestions), gradually leading the client from external to internal orientation and from an existing to a desired state.

> ...you are sitting in this chair AND you are breathing AND you can relax your muscles, that's right, AND feel comfortable AND memories can come to mind AND the feelings they bring along...

This example begins with two observable states (truisms) 'sitting in this chair' and 'breathing'. All other states are suggestions for desired states. Each time the client accepts and follows a suggestion, the desired state becomes a new current state. It can be ratified ('that's right') and utilised as a truism for the next step ('and...'). Timing is key in this process. Brooks often suggests a state (e.g. relaxation of facial muscles) when it just begins to happen. He might say: "Your facial muscles begin to smooth out". This is a three-fold message to the client:

- His explicit words say: I see what happens, I pay attention.
- His voice tone says: this is okay.
- The implication (begin to..) is: you can continue to do this.

Using serial suggestions is not always a straight line from an external observable state to an internal non-observable state. A client can go into trance and come back several times, each time going deeper. Serial suggestions can follow these movements. For the hypnotherapist, this is all about being alert and flexible. It's about observation and utilisation: the two basic principles underlying Brooks' work. In the course of a session, Brooks develops a new associational network, linking simple observations and facts to trance phenomena, resources, desired states and problem resolution. The client's limiting or destructive associational network is challenged, loosened or overruled by something more constructive and supportive.

Examples from the Spider Phobia session:

> I would like you to, kind of collect your thoughts AND think about this problem you've got.
>
> Open your eyes AND see if you can feel comfortable.
>
> Allow your eyes to close all the way AND go into a nice comfortable relaxed state.
>
> Until they just can't wait anymore AND they have to close.
>
> Just leaving you feeling nice AND comfortable AND relaxed, each time you breathe.
>
> She's gonna be very relaxed on the beach, totally relaxed AND confident AND comfortable.

Connecting paradoxical states

Adjunctive suggestions can also be used to connect states that seem to oppose each other. Here the words 'yet', 'even if', 'although' or 'even though' are used.

> You are suspicious about hypnosis YET your breathing is slowing down.
>
> And you will know what is best for you EVEN IF that is a new experience.
>
> Trance is happening EVEN THOUGH your conscious mind is very active.

Examples from the Spider Phobia session:

> You have the laser still on that cloud, EVEN THOUGH it's now down by the ground.

Contrasting different states

Finally, adjunctive suggestions can be used to contrast different states by using the word 'but'.

> Your breathing is slowing down BUT you are not in trance yet, are you?
>
> Your head is awake BUT your body is in a deep trance.

Examples from the Spider Phobia session:

> It seems to be a problem to you, having this, BUT do you really want to get rid of it altogether?
>
> As your arm starts to get a little heavier, as it starts to want to lower, BUT don't let it lower all the way down yet.

Dependent suggestions

These are suggestions[35] that are made dependent on an ongoing or expected behaviour using a subordinate clause of time (see also chapter 4). The desired behaviour is linked to a time-bound behaviour using words like 'as', 'while', 'whilst', 'when', 'before', 'after', 'whenever', 'each time', 'anytime',' once' or 'don't until'.

For example:

> AS your eyes are blinking, you can go into trance.
>
> You can begin to feel that change AS you are stretching out your hands.
>
> You can notice that sensation WHILE those hands are coming together.
>
> WHEN you open your eyes, an unexpected image will come to mind.
>
> WHENEVER the feeling comes up, it can now be welcomed.
>
> EACH TIME you breathe out, you can go deeper into trance.
>
> DON'T go into trance UNTIL that arm touches your face.

Note that the 'ongoing' process can be placed before or after the 'desired' process. Dependent suggestions not only link an ongoing and a desired behaviour, they also presuppose the ongoing behaviour.

> AS your eyes are blinking, you can go into trance.
>
> > Presupposition: your eyes are blinking.

The aspect of presupposition becomes more important if the ongoing behaviour is not observable.

> As your arms are getting heavy, you can feel more comfortable.

---

[35] Dependent suggestions are also referred to as contingent suggestions (Erickson, Rossi, & Rossi, 1976).

Presupposition: your arms are getting heavy.

The presupposition is either describing or suggesting heaviness in the arms, depending on whether the client already experiences it or not. In Ericksonian hypnotherapy, there is often an overlap between describing or suggesting a state or behaviour. Brooks regularly suggests something to a client which has just started to happen, thus linking the client's behaviour to his words.

Examples from the Spider Phobia session:

> WHILE you are doing that, I would like you to, kind of collect your thoughts.
>
> ONCE you have learned to get over it, you won't, you can't unlearn that.
>
> AS your arm starts to get heavy, you go a little deeper relaxed.
>
> DON'T allow your eyes to close all the way and go into a nice comfortable, relaxed state all the way UNTIL that hand lowers all the way down to the chair.
>
> Just leaving you feeling nice and comfortable and relaxed, EACH TIME you breathe.
>
> WHEN I lift it into the air, you'll notice it starts to become a little rigid and fixed in the air.

Correlative comparative

This is a form of linking where two comparative words are linked. Examples are: 'the more...the more...', 'the more...the less...', 'the harder...the faster…'. Some examples are:

> THE SLOWER you say this, THE STRANGER it will sound.
>
> THE MORE tense that arm becomes, THE MORE relaxed the other one will get.

A correlative comparative often used by Brooks is:

> THE HARDER you try to..., THE MORE difficult it becomes.

This is called the law of reversed effort (see Chapter 6).

Examples from the Spider Phobia session:

> THE MORE your eyelids flutter, THE EASIER it's gonna be.

THE HARDER you try to bend it, THE MORE rigid it becomes.

Cause-effect

Dependent and adjunctive suggestions are implicit links. The connection between the current and the desired state is suggested but not explicitly stated. For some clients, explicit cause-effect links work better; this is especially true of clients who use these links in their own thinking and speaking. Explicit cause-effect links employ words like 'because[36]', 'causes', 'makes', 'must be', 'leads to', 'in order to', 'by', 'so', etc.

> That particular sound will MAKE you go into trance easily.
>
> Nervousness finally LEADS TO deep trance.
>
> You learned to do this SO you can learn to do something else.

Also, if a client is in a deep trance and the conscious mind is no longer in the way, implicit links are no longer needed, and explicit ones can be more effective.

Examples from the Spider Phobia session:

> They are actually quite minor BECAUSE they are very easy to get over
>
> I'd like you to help me to help her, SO together we can both help her.
>
> He is feeling much more comfortable, BECAUSE he can trust her.

Explanatory links

Just like dependent and adjunctive links, explanatory links connect current states to desired states. In this case, the current state is kind of an explanation for the desired state:

> Nervousness is a PREREQUISITE FOR a good trance.
>
> Breathing deeply can be a GATEWAY TO deep relaxation.
>
> To choose hypnotherapy is the BEGINNING OF the resolution.

Often the current state is an emotional state, as in the first example. It can also be a physical or mental behaviour, as in the second and third examples respectively. Note that explanatory links can be literal (like 'prerequisite' or

---

[36] The word because is also used as a discourse marker at the beginning of a sentence, to loosely connect the suggestion to the previous communication or wider context.

'beginning') or metaphorical ('gateway'). Typically, on both sides of the connection, a nominalisation ('nervousness', 'trance', 'relaxation') or the gerund or infinite form of a verb ('breathing', 'to choose') is used. This allows the speaker to omit the personal pronoun (you) in the sentence making the suggestion artfully vague (see also Chapter 3).

Examples from the Spider Phobia session:

> The fluttering in your eyelids, is so CHARACTERISTIC OF a good hypnotic subject

Superseding links

Yet another way of using links is to supersede a limiting link with a stronger supporting link. Suppose a client gets nervous when thinking about a presentation he must give. If you can somehow make him laugh while thinking of the presentation, and keep him laughing for a while, a new link develops: 'idea of the presentation' – 'state of laughter'. When this link becomes strong enough, it can supersede the original link: 'idea of the presentation' – 'nervousness'. Limiting links can be superseded by eliciting any positive state that is somehow opposite to[37] and stronger than the problem state. Brooks often elicits relaxation, humour, compassion and love as powerful supportive states to replace limiting states or simply to expand the client's experiential repertoire. In the Spider Phobia session, he uses humour at the beginning to deal with the client's nervousness and to create a beginning link between the idea of spiders and positive feelings. Throughout the session, he elicits relaxation and comfort to counteract possible states of fear or panic. Towards the end, he links states of pleasure, trust and friendship to the image of a spider. All these positive states are linked to the concept and perception of spiders, either explicitly or implicitly[38], and replace or supersede the client's limiting links.

---

[37] It does not need to be the formal opposite of the problem state, just the subjective opposite for the client.

[38] Implicit linking occurs by experiencing these states in the context of spider phobia therapy.

Linking trance phenomena

Milton Erickson considered trance phenomena a normal life experience that happens in certain circumstances. Time distortion can happen during a wonderful party (time flies) or during a boring lecture (time drags). Catalepsy can occur when we are startled by a loud bang, and we are literally scared stiff. Trance phenomena happen all the time as a result of everyday experiences. Conversely, we can use hypnosis to elicit trance phenomena as examples for life experiences. The sense of comfort in trance can represent working, relating or living comfortably. The trance experience of amnesia can prove that the client can forget 'things', i.e. negative memories. Time distortion can help a client to contract painful times and expand those of comfort. Trance phenomena can be explicitly linked to daily life by suggestions like:

> This sensation of calmness will occur by surprise when you need it. It will be interesting to discover how moments of pain will seem so short whereas times of comfort will seem so long.

Even without these suggestions, experiencing a trance phenomenon as part of a hypnotherapy session implies that they are relevant for the client's life[39]. In the Spider Phobia session, Brooks observes the phenomenon of fluttering eyelids and links it to:

> being a good hypnotic subject (meaning)
>
> making changes happen (consequence)
>
> making them happen automatically, easily and comfortably (consequence)

He also equates the phenomenon of the catalepsy of the client's arm with her strength and defines it as proof of her power, his power and the power of hypnosis. The trance phenomenon of dissociation is implicitly used as an example of being separate from the image of a spider and of being in control of the perception of it.

---

[39] As opposed to trance phenomena during stage hypnosis, which are implied to occur on stage only.

Frames

The aspect of splitting and linking is closely related to the concept of frames. A client's problem is always experienced within a certain context. Even when a client thinks the problem occurs always and everywhere, this is unlikely to be true; it probably happens in certain situations, and with certain people, i.e. it is context dependent. Apart from the external context, clients have internal contexts (frames) around their experiences. They create mental frames around concrete observations. The concrete part of an experience is the current sensory input, i.e. what you see, hear, sense, taste or smell at the present moment. The conceptual part consists of various thoughts, ideas and beliefs organised in mental frames. A frame can be seen as a pair of coloured spectacles: it determines how you see the world around you. There are frames of name, time, cause, meaning and intention; and all offer different ways of interpreting an object, event or process. Since this book is about treating fear of spiders, let's look at the frames that might be activated when seeing a spider. A little baby will see a spider without any frames. The spider is simply an image with no meaning. The baby might respond with a natural sense of curiosity and tendency to touch it. It has a frameless experience of encountering a spider[40]. For an adult who is not afraid of spiders, the observation of a spider in the kitchen cupboard might activate frames and related thoughts like:

- Name: this is a spider.
- Meaning: this means the cupboard should be cleaned more often.
- Intention: I need to remove the spider.

From these frames, the person might have a neutral emotional response and the behavioural response of removing the spider. Now let's look at the possible frames of a person with a spider phobia upon seeing one in the kitchen cupboard. The concrete external part of the experience is the same: the image of a spider. The activated frames, however, will be much more extensive and might involve frames of:

- Time: how long has it been there?

[40] In the Spider Phobia session, an image of a baby relating to a spider is actually used as a resource.

- Cause: how did it get here?
- Expectation: it could jump on my body.
- Meaning: this is dangerous.
- Intention: I need to get out of here.

These frames will provoke a much stronger emotional (fear) and behavioural response (running away). Unfortunately, the framing of this experience doesn't stop there. The feeling of fear and the act of running are framed as well. Some examples are:

- Judgment: being afraid of spiders is *stupid*.
- Social: people will laugh at me.

After several encounters with a spider, the 'process' of feeling fear and running away will gradually become a 'thing' with a name: a spider phobia. The activated frames will involve beliefs, rather than just thoughts. For example:

- Naming: this is a phobia.
- Time: I have had this phobia for many years.
- Cause: I have inherited it from my mother.
- Generalisation: there can be spiders anywhere.
- Meaning: having this phobia means I am in constant danger.
- Consequence: I can't go to unknown places.
- Control: I can't change my phobic response.
- Identity: I am a phobic.
- Intention: I want to get rid of this phobia.

Any of these frames can play a crucial role in maintaining the problem or solving it. Some frames might need to be addressed before others can be tackled. Suppose the cause-frame includes the belief "my phobia is genetic". This frame might prevent any psychotherapeutic change since the client believes the problem is not psychological. Links, in the form of beliefs, can occur within a frame, e.g.:

- Time: I've had this phobia for *many years*, so I'll *always* have it.

or across frames, e.g.:

- Cause – time: this problem is *hereditary*, so I'll *always* have it.
- Social – identity: *no one else* is afraid of spiders; I must *be a chicken*.

Note that frames in themselves are not positive or negative; they are just a way of looking at something. It is the choice of frame or its content (ideas, beliefs) which makes it either limiting or supporting. Reframing is a technique of changing frames and the ideas they involve. This technique is described in Chapter 6.

Non-Attachment as an approach to therapy

People's ideas, beliefs and frames of reference can cause many problems and limitations. It isn't just the limiting nature of thoughts or beliefs, but also the client's level of attachment to those thoughts that play an important role. As a Buddhist, Brooks has embraced the principle of non-attachment and applied it to therapy. According to this principle, all human suffering is caused by attachment to things, ideas, beliefs, roles, status, fame etc. Non-attachment, on the other hand, is considered the way to inner peace and happiness. During his years in Thailand Brooks developed a powerful technique which integrates hypnotherapeutic and Buddhist principles. He calls this approach Non Attachment Therapy (NAT). It can be used with any problems involving a negative feeling or emotion. The result is a fast release of the limiting beliefs underlying a problem, a feeling of non-attachment with respect to a problem context, followed by a deep sense of freedom to move forward and achieve whatever life goals were being inhibited by the problem. Brooks uses NAT as a stand-alone therapy, however, the principles of non-attachment are at the very foundation of his unique approach to Compassionate Ericksonian hypnotherapy.

Chapter 6: Various Ericksonian Techniques

With a career spanning more than 50 years, Milton Erickson developed a vast array of techniques, many of which have found their way into modern hypnotherapy, NLP, Solution Focused Therapy, Systems Therapy and various other fields. This chapter will focus on those techniques used in the Spider Phobia session described in this book, the main ones being hypnotic desensitisation and double dissociation.

V/K (Double) Dissociation

Dissociation in Ericksonian hypnotherapy refers to the separation of two experiences. This can be the dissociation between the conscious and the unconscious mind, between thinking and doing or between seeing and feeling. The latter is called Visual/Kinaesthetic (V/K) dissociation. It means the feelings of a memory or experience are separated from the images. The opposite of dissociation is association, which means being engaged in the experience with all your senses: images, sounds, feelings etc. Full association of a past experience means reliving it as if it is happening again. This is actually what happens if a person with a phobia thinks of or is confronted with the feared object. V/K dissociation can be used to look at yourself (your former self) in a negative experience. As such, you can see the experience without having the feelings. A double V/K dissociation means you are looking at your current self, who is looking at your former self in the negative experience. Where the problem of a phobia is association, its solution is dissociation or double dissociation. The standard NLP phobia cure (Bandler, 1985) (O'Connor, 2001) uses an imaginary movie theatre for double dissociation and leads the client with direct instructions. By contrast, Brooks begins by inducing trance, utilises the client's favourite place for double dissociation and combines this technique with hypnotic desensitisation. He indirectly and playfully leads the client through the procedure, subtly following and utilising her responses.

Hypnotic desensitisation

A technique often used to cure phobias is desensitisation. Using this method, the client is gradually exposed to the object of fear while experiencing relaxation. In (Cognitive) Behavioural Therapy, the client is usually exposed to real-life situations (in vivo desensitisation) and consciously learns a relaxation technique to counter the fear. In hypnotherapy, the client is exposed to an imaginary object of fear. In trance, he or she visualises or even hallucinates the spider, snake, small space or whatever it is that causes the fear. The advantage is that the hypnotherapist has control over the situation and can use trance phenomena like relaxation, dissociation or time distortion to counteract any possible fear. In the Spider Phobia session, Brooks uses relaxation and double dissociation to prevent the client's fear from occurring. He also applies a stepwise approach of desensitisation using two different modalities: digital and visual. He first has her visualise the letters of the word 'spider', one at a time. Using indirect suggestion, he then lets her see a still image of a spider at a distance that gradually turns into a moving picture that comes closer. Brooks not only desensitises her fear of spiders, he also redefines spiders from dangerous creatures to innocent friends. As such, she can, not only have a different behavioural response to spiders but also a different cognitive concept about them. At the end of the session, Brooks gives the client the posthypnotic suggestion of finding friends (spiders) in the building, thereby bringing the success of the therapy into the outer world.

Ratification

Brooks frequently confirms and ratifies the client's words or behaviour. He does this verbally by saying 'yes', 'okay', 'that's right' or with other words that express confirmation. He also does this nonverbally by nodding his head, smiling, opening his hands or making a confirming sound like 'hmmm'. Ratifying the client's behaviour is a way of letting the client know that he or she is doing okay. It is a way of inviting the client to express him or herself more. Clients are often worried about not being able to go into trance or not being able to explain or solve their problem. They are afraid of appearing stupid or weird. Ratifying everything they say or do can, gradually, take away these worries and enable them to open up, go into trance and solve their problem.

A special form of ratification has to do with trance phenomena. When clients come for hypnotherapy, they will expect to be put into a trance. However, they might not recognise trance when it occurs, because they don't know what to look for or because of false ideas about it. In which case it is necessary to point out trance phenomena as they happen. The hypnotherapist might say, "Your blink rate is changing" or "Those fingers are now moving all by themselves". A very convincing trance phenomenon is the inability to perform an otherwise easy task, e.g. opening your eyes. After eye closure, the hypnotherapist can say, "You can *try* to open your eyes and *notice that you can't*". Other examples are the inability to move an arm (catalepsy), feel a hand (anaesthesia) or remember your age or name (amnesia).

Complimenting

Clients may have doubts about their ability to go into trance, or to take therapeutic steps and integrate these changes into their lives. Complementing the client is a good way to help them overcome their doubts and strengthen their self-confidence. A direct way of complimenting is using statements like "you are doing fine", "well done" or "good job", often used in everyday life, especially with children. In hypnotherapy, it is effective for clients who can easily accept direct compliments. Some people, however, have learned to reject or disqualify compliments and so with them, you can use indirect ways of giving compliments, e.g. by embedding them in linguistic structures. For example:

> As a colleague of mine would say: "Well done".
>
> I'm almost tempted to say, "Good job".

Alternatively, you can use statements that imply a compliment. For example:

> Statement: Congratulations on taking this step.
>
> Implied compliment: Taking this step is valuable/important.
>
> Statement: Thank you for joining us here.
>
> Implied compliment: Joining us here is valuable/important.

In *1001 Solution Focused Questions* (Bannink, 2010) two other ways of complimenting a client are described.

The first one is asking competence questions like:

"How did you manage to do that?"

"How did you know you need to change?"

By answering such a question, the client creates a self-compliment, often without being aware of doing so. Even if the client answers a competence question with "I don't know", the implied compliment will be picked up by the unconscious. In Ericksonian hypnotherapy, competence questions are usually not directed to the conscious mind, and no answer is expected. They are posed with a playful and wondering voice tone and body language to appeal to the unconscious mind. The implied message is: you did something well, and it was your unconscious that did it.

The second way is the so-called positive character interpretation. Here the client's behaviour (positive or negative) is interpreted as an expression of a positive identity or personality. For example:

Positive behaviour: facing your biggest fear

Compliment: "You must be *a courageous person* to face your biggest fear"

Negative behaviour: worry too much about daughter

Compliment: "You must be *a caring mother* to worry so much about your daughter"

Brooks sometimes uses a special form of this type of compliment by defining the client's response as evidence of being 'a good hypnotic subject'.

In the Spider Phobia session, he mainly uses direct compliments. He can do this because the client has an external reference, trusts his opinion and easily accepts compliments. However, he does use some implied compliments, positive character interpretations and competence questions. For example:

You are doing very well.

Well done.

Congratulations on getting here now.

Thank you for coming all the way up here.

The fluttering in your eyelids is so characteristic of a good hypnotic subject.

How did you do that?

Age regression/revivification

Although Ericksonian hypnotherapy is often present and future-oriented, Brooks uses age regression when he considers it appropriate and useful. In a true age regression, the client experiences him or herself to be younger and actually believes this to be the case. Full regression requires a deep trance in which the client becomes totally unaware of external reality. A milder version of regression is revivification. Here, the client can see him or herself as being younger while being aware of his or her true age. This experience is much easier to attain and can be reached in a light trance. Revivification is a state somewhere between a deep trance, full regression and a normal waking state. The Spider Phobia session described in this book contains some elements of revivification at the beginning of the session, but regression/revivification is not the overall technique here.

Visualisation

A common technique in hypnotherapy is visualisation. This means the client is encouraged, by suggestion, to see something in his or her mind's eye. A visualisation includes images, but also sounds, feelings, smells and tastes; it involves all the five senses. Visualisation can be used for trance induction, memory retrieval, resource elicitation, goal setting or any other therapeutic step. In traditional hypnosis and many other therapeutic fields, clients are given direct instructions for visualisation, e.g. "Imagine a beautiful landscape". In Ericksonian hypnotherapy, visualisation is often attained indirectly. This can be done by employing indirect suggestions like "I wonder what you are beginning to see in your mind's eye". It can also be done by telling stories or by using metaphors or analogies, e.g. "When I was a boy I lived on a big farm near a forest..." A visualisation can be passive in the sense that the hypnotherapist describes an imaginary scene or journey and leads the client through it. It can also be interactive in the sense that therapist and client co-create an imaginary journey. In the Spider Phobia session detailed in this book, Brooks creates an extensive and interactive visualisation for problem resolution, including various techniques of association, dissociation, hypnotic desensitisation and reframing. He utilises the client's ability to visualise and starts the journey on her favourite place: the beach.

Using metaphors and symbols

Brooks uses metaphors extensively, creating stories that somehow match the client's experience. The client's situation or problem is translated to a metaphorical context where a certain figure, character or person has a similar problem and solves it. Metaphors must be isomorphic in the sense that they somehow resemble the client's situation, problem, experience, goal etc. (Gordon, 1978). The time, place, characters, and events of the metaphor, however, can be completely different to the client's real life. In fact, they should be different enough for the client not to relate it directly (consciously) to him or herself. The story should be interesting or acceptable for the conscious mind, while the unconscious picks up hidden messages. Just like visualisations, metaphors can be passive or interactive with respect to the client. A passive metaphor is simply a story told by the hypnotherapist. An interactive metaphor is developed in a dialogue between the hypnotherapist and the client. The difference between a visualisation and a metaphor is that in the latter, the client is replaced by the main character of the story. In a visualisation, it is the client himself who experiences the story or journey. A metaphor can be started by the hypnotherapist, for example, "Your situation reminds me of..." or by a figure of speech from the client, for example, "I feel like I'm carrying the world on my shoulders". As a hypnotherapist, you can utilise such a figure of speech by taking it literally, e.g. "Which part of the world doesn't belong on your shoulders?" As such, you can start an interactive metaphor that can be visualised in the client's mind, acted out physically in the session or turned into a therapeutic task, e.g. "I want you to go to the gym, and enjoy lifting various weights and putting them down".

In the Spider Phobia session, Brooks creates the story (metaphor) of Harry the spider. It is not a typical metaphor with a different context and different characters, but one utilising the same characters with their roles reversed. The spider becomes the frightened, captured victim that is freed by the client. Freeing the scared and locked-up spider means freeing her younger self. The image of a spider —which was the source of her fear— has become the key to resolving her fear. This is a neat example of utilising the problem to create a solution.

Metaphors can be verbal, as described above, or they can be nonverbal. A nonverbal metaphor is a gesture, movement or facial expression that expresses a message from the unconscious mind. Often these expressions happen while the client is telling his or her story or answering a question and may support or contradict the words. Any incongruity between conscious words and unconscious body language is interesting for the hypnotherapist because this reveals an area of internal conflict. Also, physical symptoms like pain or tension can be seen as a metaphor for the underlying problem. These are called organic metaphors.

Symbols are similar to metaphors in that they represent something else. They are, however, concrete objects or representations, standing for abstract ideas or concepts. In daily life, people use all kind of symbols. The heart, for example, is for many people a symbol of love whereas a bird may stand for freedom. In hypnotherapy, symbols can be used to represent the client's problem, resources or solution. In the spider phobia session, Brooks utilises the client's rings and the stones in them as symbols for light and a key as a symbol to power and freedom.

Analogy

Brooks also uses many analogies, telling stories about other people who have had similar problems or issues. These other people can be clients, friends, relatives or even the hypnotherapist himself. Especially effective are analogies about previous clients who have experienced comparable problems and successfully overcome them. These analogies indirectly suggest that the problem can be solved and that the therapist knows how to do this. In the Spider Phobia session, Brooks does this at the beginning; he talks about a former client with a similar problem. The indirect messages being: 'I have worked with this kind of problem before', 'it is not hereditary', 'it is a learned problem'. A little later he asks a previous client, who happens to be in the audience, to share her parallel story. This is an active analogy, which is even more powerful than a told one. The messages here are 'I have worked with someone with this problem in this same chair' and 'the work was successful'. Like embedded and interspersed suggestions, analogies and metaphors are used indirectly and frequently by Brooks to put across relevant messages.

Anchoring

Anchoring is an NLP technique (O'Connor, 2001) that stems mainly from Erickson's work. An anchor is a link between a trigger —e.g. an image, sound, word or touch— and a certain state or response. For example, a touch on the shoulder often elicits a state of comfort in the recipient. Links between sensory experience and an internal state are created all the time in daily life, often because the two occur simultaneously. You associate a song with a certain mood, simply because it was once played when you were in that mood. In hypnotherapy and NLP, anchors are created deliberately to give a 'handle' for eliciting desired states. In the Spider Phobia session, Brooks anchors the client's state of comfort and relaxation to a touch on her shoulder. Similarly, those same states are anchored to the words *comfortable* and *relaxed.*

Scaling

Scaling is a technique of measuring something within a certain range, e.g. from 0 to 10. It can be used to measure the severity of a problem, therapeutic progress or a client's motivation or confidence. Scaling is a standard technique in Solution Focused Therapy (De Shazer & Dolan, 2007) and in EMDR (Shapiro, 2001), and it is often used in hypnotherapy. How serious is the problem? How bad has it ever been? How did you manage to reduce the symptom from 10 to 8? How much confidence do you have in being able to solve this? These are all questions that help the client a get a concrete handle on the problem. Scaling helps break down the therapeutic process into manageable steps. The question is no longer "How do I solve my problem?" but "How do I get from 10 to 8 or from 8 to 7?" Scaling gives both client and hypnotherapist insight into the progress and effectiveness of the therapy. Some clients tend to focus on the things that have not been solved yet and forget about the steps they have made. Scaling reminds them of their progress, encourages them be proud and to keep going. A problem severity scale can run from 0 to 10 or from 0 to 100 as long as you do it consistently. Alternatively, you can use a solution scale, with 0 signifying the problem at its worst and 10 meaning it is completely solved. Scaling someone's experience is not a scientific measurement like taking someone's temperature or blood pressure. It is a subjective estimate that both indicates and influences the client's experience. In the Spider Phobia session, Brooks asks the client to scale her fear between 1 and 10. She says it's 11. Choosing a number beyond the scale shows the severity of her problem but it also gives it a humorous touch. Brooks utilises her answer for indirect suggestion. Overtly he 'explains' to the audience, "We're gonna bring that right down, so she feels perfectly fine". Covertly he is 'suggesting' to her that she should bring her fear down and feel fine. At the end of the session, when she is back from the trance, he asks her to think of spiders again and scale her fear. It has gone down from 11 to 0. It is an enormous shift in her experience. Brooks however realises that the number 0 is not an objective fact and no guarantee that her fear has entirely disappeared. He uses scaling here not just to test but also to have her experience and realise the change. 'Realising' the shift is one of the final steps of therapy. The same goes for Brooks congratulating her, having her take ownership of the therapeutic change and sending her off to find spiders. He is using every opportunity to solidify therapeutic success.

Future Pacing

Future pacing means orienting the client towards the future with respect to the desired or achieved changes. The client can see (dissociated) or experience (associated) him or herself in all kinds of future situations with the new behaviour/ideas/beliefs and evaluate their usefulness and validity. As such, future pacing is a built-in ecology check[41], i.e. it is a test of whether or not the therapeutic change is desirable and appropriate. It can happen at any point in therapy: before, during or after an intervention. In NLP, future pacing is usually done explicitly, and the client is asked to consciously imagine future situations. Brooks usually does it implicitly, using various indirect suggestions, metaphors and tasks. Using vague words, he describes possible future consequences and systemic effects while monitoring the client's responses. At the start of the Spider Phobia session, Brooks talks about the client and her family being free of the problem. At the end of the session, he uses two kinds of future pacing; Firstly, he gives the client the task of finding spiders (now defined as friends) in the building, secondly, he has her think of her baby daughter and imagine the

41 Ecology is a term used in NLP for the study of the consequences of a change for the client's future and social system.

positive consequences for her. As such, he helps her carry the changes of the session into her future and into her family system.

Creating amnesia

To keep a client from blocking, disturbing or even destroying the unconscious changes, Brooks often creates amnesia for the trance experience. Interestingly, in many therapeutic schools the client is encouraged to be aware of the changes, remember them and apply them consciously. In Ericksonian hypnotherapy we do the opposite. Brooks helps the client to forget what happened in the session so the changes can take effect unconsciously. He uses various techniques for amnesia, depending on the client and the stage of the session. During the session, he often uses an amnesia gap by using the same word or phrase before and after a suggestion. Sometimes he distracts the conscious mind after a suggestion by quickly changing the subject or asking an irrelevant question. Creating amnesia for the entire trance experience can be accomplished in various ways:

- By referring to the beginning of the session when the client opens his or her eyes. This can be done by saying "Hi" (as if you just met) or referring to a topic that was mentioned in the beginning.
- By immediately distracting the client when he or she comes out of hypnosis, e.g. by drawing attention to something completely unrelated.
- By suggesting that the client should 'try' to remember 'everything' about the session, implying that this will be difficult or impossible.
- By using a metaphor for forgetting, e.g. "Sometimes when you wake up, you know you had a dream, but you forgot what it was about".
- By bringing the client back very quickly.

In the Spider Phobia session, Brooks uses both the first technique —he says "Hi there" — and the second one, when he talks about her beautiful eyes. However, there is no need for complete amnesia here as the client has been very responsive throughout the session and, after the trance, she can stay with the experience without much conscious involvement.

Law of reversed effort

Brooks often uses the so-called law of reversed effort (Erickson, Rossi, & Rossi, 1976). This law states that the act of trying implies difficulty and the harder you try to do something, the more difficult it becomes. It is a paradoxical principle in which we instruct the conscious mind to 'try' and do something and expect it to fail. This is an elegant way of utilising the conscious mind's need for control. The conscious mind is told to (try and) do what it wants to do anyway, while the unconscious picks up the implication of difficulty and counteracts the conscious effort. So, trying to open your eyes usually results in being unable to open them. The law of reversed effort is also a way of proving the power of hypnosis. Clients often say things like, "I was amazed that I really could not open my eyes!" It ratifies their trance experience. Furthermore, the law of reversed effort can be used for amnesia ('try to remember what happened') or for compounding a therapeutic result ('try to feel that old fear'). In the Spider Phobia session, Brooks uses an extended version of the law of reversed effort towards the end. He induces arm catalepsy and encourages her to 'try' to bend her arm. He repeats this suggestion several times and with variations of the message "the harder you try, the more rigid it becomes".

Moving the client around

A well-known Ericksonian technique is to constantly move/juggle the client around, mentally, emotionally or physically. This is another way of depotentiating the conscious mind and decreasing conscious control. The client can be moved around with respect to:

- sensory systems: visual, auditory, kinaesthetic, olfactory and gustatory.
- time orientation: past, present and future.
- location: having the client move, walk, change seats etc.
- contexts: therapeutic, work, home, leisure activity.
- states of association and dissociation.
- external and internal experience.
- physical posture and position.

All these ways of moving the client around can help him or her to let go of conscious control and allow for unconscious processes to happen. In the Spider Phobia session, Brooks doesn't need to do this a lot because the client is very responsive. In the first part of the session, he goes back and forth between talking to her and talking to the audience, giving suggestions, and asking for factual information, associating her with her fear and dissociating her from it. After a short while she is in full rapport with him, follows his lead, and no further depotentiating of her conscious is needed.

Using the negative

Brooks uses negative formulations with words like 'not', 'can't', 'don't', 'nothing', 'stop' and 'without' in his communication. Often, this is a way of matching, anticipating or discharging negativity, doubt or resistance on the part of the client. A simple example of this is repeating or using the client's negative nominalisations or verbs like 'fear', 'crisis', 'to hate', 'to block' etc. or their negative statements like "I can't do this" or "I will never be happy". Brooks usually doesn't repeat these words literally, as is done in NLP, he will utilise a client's negatives more subtly and indirectly. In the Spider Phobia session, the client uses the word 'scared' a few times at the start. Brooks utilises this word later in the imagined story of the 'scared' spider. Other examples of using the negative were discussed in previous chapters:

> Negative embedded suggestion: <u>Don't</u> go into trance.
>
> Negative embedded suggestion with implication: <u>Don't</u> go into trance yet.
>
> Tag question: It is possible, <u>isn't it</u>?

Sometimes the negative is used to repeat a positive suggestion with a negative formulation. The client can then respond to whichever formulation fits best.

> You can experience <u>more</u> relaxation, <u>less</u> tension.

Obviously, the negative can be used to deny what the other person says, as is often done in daily life. In hypnotherapy, if we want to deny something the client thinks or says we tend not to do it directly but within an indirect suggestion, metaphor or analogy. In the Spider Phobia session, Brooks denies the client's belief that her phobia is hereditary by using the analogy of a former client who had a Daddy Longlegs phobia. He firmly refutes the previous client's belief of it being hereditary, thereby indirectly denying that of the current client's.

Examples of using the negative in the Spider Phobia session:

> But it is <u>not</u> hereditary, it's <u>impossible</u>. (denying within an analogy)

Don't let it lower all the way down yet. (negative embedded suggestion with implication)

You feel okay, do you not? (tag)

Feel comfortable and not scared. (positive and negative formulation)

Frustrating response

In Ericksonian hypnotherapy, we often suggest that the client hold back a desired response, both in trance induction and in therapy. Brooks might say something like, "don't go all the way down yet" to keep the client from going into a deep trance. The desired response is frustrated, which increases the motivation to have it. Furthermore, the word 'yet' implies that the client will 'go all the way down' eventually. Holding back the desired state also validates the client's current state. Don't go 'there' implies that it is okay to be 'here'. Frustrating a response also gives the hypnotherapist an opportunity to introduce a condition for the desired state: "This arm will not go down until your unconscious is ready to go into a deep trance". The desired response of lowering the arm is frustrated and made dependent upon 'readiness to go into a deep trance'. Since the arm will go down at some point because of gravity or fatigue, going into a deep trance becomes very compelling.

An example from the induction phase of the Spider Phobia session:

> As your arm starts to get a little heavier, as it starts to want to lower, but don't let it lower all the way down yet because when it starts to lower, I want you to go deeply and deeply relaxed, each time it lowers a little at a time, deeper and slowly, let your whole body relax.

Opposite direction

Milton Erickson sometimes used the technique of instructing the client to go in the opposite direction to the desired goal. For example, if someone wanted to lose weight, he would instruct him or her to gain weight first. Changing a symptom in any direction proves that the client has control over it and change is possible. Clients generally expect a therapist to help them go in the right direction. Suggesting a change in the 'wrong' direction is, therefore, confusing for the conscious mind and thus reduces conscious control. Going in the opposite direction can also provoke a counter-reaction in the client; an urge to oppose the suggestion of the therapist and move in the desired direction. Whether the client follows or opposes the move in the 'wrong' direction, the result is therapeutic. In the Spider Phobia session, Brooks uses this technique when he has the client move a visualised cloud (which serves as a projection screen for a spider image) farther away before bringing it closer.

Repetition

Brooks will repeat words, phrases, sentences and ideas. This is a way of compounding a suggestion or idea, and it increases the chance that the client will pick it up and realise it. In Ericksonian hypnotherapy, words are not simply repeated in the same way, as is often the case in traditional hypnosis. Brooks will repeat a certain word, a number of times, while varying his voice tone or gestures. He might also repeat an idea using synonyms for certain keywords. He will say something indirectly and then directly, metaphorically and then literally. A suggestion can be given when the client is in trance and it can be repeated when he or she is out of trance. Repeating the same thing in different ways is a way of avoiding conscious resistance, stopping the client thinking, "Why is he saying this again?" and taking conscious control. When the client is in a deep enough trance, the conscious mind is no longer active, and words can simply be repeated as they are. In the Spider Phobia session, Brooks uses a lot of repetition. At the beginning, he repeats the idea of the client's fear being a learned problem, several times. In the course of the induction, he uses words like 'deeper', 'relaxed' and 'comfortable' repeatedly. Towards the end of the session, the idea of her not hurting Harry the spider[42] is reiterated in various wordings.

Reframing

In chapter 5 we discussed the nature of frames and the type of frames that exist. Reframing is the technique of changing mental frames and the ideas and beliefs they involve. Two basic forms are content reframing and context reframing. Content reframing involves challenging or changing the content of a frame. For example:

---

[42] The idea of her not hurting Harry implies she could hurt him, which in turn implies she is in control.

Client: Being afraid means being weak (meaning-frame)

Therapist: I would say that being afraid means being human

Client: I think my fear is hereditary (cause-frame)

Therapist: Are you sure it's hereditary?

Context reframing involves putting a negative feeling or behaviour in a context where it is positive. An example would be:

Client: I'm scared of spiders; I run when I see one.

Therapist: In the case of a Black Widow spider, being scared and running is probably a healthy response.

Besides these basic forms, reframing can involve enlarging a frame or switching frames. An example of this would be:

Client: I have had this fear for 10 years. (time-frame)

Therapist: What is 10 years in a lifetime? (enlarging time-frame)

You have had this for 10 years and now it is time to let it go. (switching from time-frame to intention-frame)

In the Spider Phobia session, Brooks applies various forms of reframing. In the first few minutes of the session, he seeds the idea of harmlessness and begins to reframe the meaning of spiders from dangerous to harmless creatures. He also reframes the possible 'cause' of her fear, from inherited to learned. The client's 'intention' towards spiders changes from avoiding them to finding them and becoming friends with them. Her intention towards her phobia is redefined and enlarged from "her getting rid of" to "her and her family being free from it". Within the identity-frame, she moves from being a bad mother who is teaching her child to be phobic, to being a good mother who is blessing her child with many gifts. From a systemic point of view, Brooks helps her to make a shift within three related frames ('time', 'identity' and 'significant other') from her past —being the 'daughter' of her 'mother'— to her 'future': being the 'mother' of her 'child'. More about reframing can be found in NLP literature (Dilts R. B., 1999) (Hall & Bodenhamer, 1997).

Keeping part of the problem

A typical Ericksonian technique is to suggest that the client keeps a part of the problem. In most therapeutic orientations, the client is encouraged and supported to fully let go of the problem. Brooks often encourages his clients to keep a certain aspect of their problem. There are several reasons for doing this. It implies there is something good about the problem. This makes sense because most problems have a positive side, although the client does not always realise this. Furthermore, giving permission to keep part of a problem takes away the pressure of having to solve it completely. Losing the problem entirely can create a sense of emptiness or even loss of identity, especially if the symptom is severe and has existed for a long time. Keeping part of the problem gives the client something to hold on to, while he or she gets accustomed to different ways of thinking, feeling and behaving. The response of a client to the suggestion of keeping part of the problem can vary. He or she might feel relieved and accept the suggestion, choosing to keep some aspect of the problem for a while or forever. The client can also reject the suggestion. In this case, it may actually motivate him or her to solve the problem completely. Both responses — accepting or rejecting the idea of keeping a part of the problem— are therapeutically valuable. The client is in a double bind. In the Spider Phobia session, Brooks asks the client, "Do you really want to get rid of it altogether?" This is an indirect suggestion of keeping a part of her fear. She rejects this suggestion: "altogether, clearly."

Distraction

In Ericksonian hypnotherapy, the client is often distracted from suggestions that have been made. Actually, it is the conscious mind that is distracted so that the unconscious can accept and utilise the suggestion. Brooks might use distraction at any point during a session, but it is especially useful during the first and last parts. At the beginning, Brooks seeds ideas, which are developed later in the session, and he wants to keep the client from consciously analysing or rejecting these ideas. At the end of a session, when the client comes out of trance, distraction can be used to create amnesia for parts of the session or all of it. In the middle of a session, distraction can be used if the client comes out of trance and becomes too consciously involved. A client can be distracted in several ways; Verbally by changing the subject, asking irrelevant questions or giving a cognitive task; Visually by unexpected gestures or facial expressions or by changes in posture or position; Kinaesthetically by touching the client's shoulder, lifting their hand or any other touch or movement that is safe and ethical. Distraction is not only used to divert the client's attention from a suggestion that has just been given, used at the beginning of a session, but it can also be a way of depotentiating the conscious mind, deepening trance and laying the groundwork for therapeutic change. At the beginning of the Spider Phobia session, Brooks uses distraction several times, asking the client irrelevant questions after planting a suggestion. At the end, he distracts her conscious mind by saying she has beautiful eyes. Actually, this is not just distraction but also a way of complimenting her (see previous paragraph in this chapter on complimenting).

Pattern intervention

A key technique in Ericksonian hypnotherapy is pattern intervention, which involves the utilisation of, or change to, a client's pattern of behaving or thinking. Problems are considered to follow a certain pattern that includes thoughts, images, feelings and actions. Utilising or changing these can solve the problem. Psychodynamically-oriented therapists may argue that this does not solve the underlying cause and therefore the problem is bound to come back. Erickson believed that limiting patterns often remain through habituation, even though the cause has long been extinguished. A person once bitten by a dog might avoid dogs out of habit and therefore remain afraid, even though the traumatic memory has faded. Even if the cause still exists as a vivid, emotionally loaded memory, pattern intervention can work. Brooks considers a symptom and its cause to be part of a present representation. As such, pattern intervention can change this representation and resolve the symptom and its cause. Bill O'Hanlon has described various forms of pattern intervention; these include changes of time, place, frequency and order, intensity of occurrence, the addition or removal of steps and the replacement of the existing pattern with a different one (O'Hanlon, 1987). Pattern intervention can take place hypnotically during a session or in the form of a task. The client in the Spider Phobia session has a pattern of checking places to avoid fearful encounters with spiders. Brooks replaces this pattern with the task of checking places in the building to create joyful encounters with spiders.

Seeding

Seeding is a technique used by Erickson, either for trance induction, eliciting trance phenomena like amnesia or for therapeutic intervention. According to Zeig, seeding can be defined as activating an intended target by presenting an earlier hint (Zeig & Gilligan, 1990). It means planting an idea into someone's mind to be built on later. In psychology, this technique is called priming, and many experiments have been done on the thoughts, feelings and behaviours of people who have been primed with a certain image, sound or idea. In literature, seeding is called foreshadowing and is used by the author to hint at what is to come. In Ericksonian hypnotherapy, seeding is used to work towards a certain response, behaviour or belief. In his book 'Uncommon Therapy' Jay Haley wrote:

> "In his hypnotic inductions, Erickson likes to 'seed' or establish certain ideas and later build upon them. He will emphasise certain ideas in the beginning of the interchange so that later if he wants to achieve a certain response, he has already laid the groundwork for that response." (Haley, 1973)

In the Spider Phobia session, Brooks seeds the idea of 'harmlessness' at the beginning of the session with a suggestion about the audience: "They are quite *harmless*". Later, during the visualisation, he seeds the idea of her problem fading away with his suggestion about the word 'spider': "Let me know when it's just *faded away* into the cloud."

Nonverbal techniques

Doing Ericksonian hypnotherapy means communicating on multiple levels and using both verbal and nonverbal techniques. Brooks is an expert in both channels of communication. Verbal communication means being artfully vague, being indirect and using implication and linking. All of this has been discussed in the previous chapters. Nonverbal communication includes everything 'except' words; it consists not only of gestures, movements, actions, facial expressions, posture and breathing, but also voice tone, inflection, timbre, pitch and volume. Let's look at some of the nonverbal skills Brooks typically uses.

Breathing

The client's breathing is an important behaviour that can be utilised for induction and therapy. Changes in breathing frequency and depth can be signs of beginning trance. It can be utilised by mentioning it, matching it or by synchronising suggestions to the client's breathing rhythm. I (JvB) often use breathing as an example of something that can be 'done' consciously but usually 'happens' unconsciously. Breathing also has a symbolic value. It is a source of life, something that literally occurs and must occur from the moment you are born until the moment you die. Physically, breathing is used to inhale oxygen and to exhale carbon dioxide. Metaphorically, it can be used to inhale positive energy, strength, love etc. and to exhale negative energy in the form of fatigue, frustration etc. The in-breath is often associated with getting ready for action whereas the out-breath is associated with relaxation. All these associations of breathing can be used in hypnotherapy. Brooks usually matches his own breathing with the client's breathing. This is a way of bringing himself (kinaesthetically) into the same state and rhythm as the client. It is also a way of letting the client know (auditorily) that breathing is important and that he is right there with him or her.

Analogue marking

Analogue marking is a technique where the therapist emphasises part of his communication nonverbally to alert the unconscious mind to it. Analogue is the counterpart of digital, which in hypnotherapy translates to verbal. Analogue communication includes everything but the words spoken. So, it is about aspects of the voice like volume, pitch, tone, rhythm and pauses. It also includes physical expressions like gestures, movements, facial expressions, changes in posture and touch. The term analogue marking usually refers to marking out embedded or interspersed suggestions. A typical example is an embedded suggestion with the actual command being emphasised:

> It is very interesting to ***discover these possibilities***.

Brooks also uses analogue marking to separate different times in the client's life. He sometimes directs his voice behind the client when he refers to the past and in front when he refers to the future:

> So you can *leave behind those memories* and *move ahead to new experiences.*

The same counts for separating different locations in a visualised experience. In the Spider Phobia session, he projects his voice upwards when he talks about a cloud up there.

Vocal techniques

Brooks uses various techniques with his voice that are also part of the repertoire of singers, actors and comedians. He plays with voice tone, volume, pitch, inflection, rhythm and pauses to influence his clients. Some examples of these are:

- Speaking softly to induce, deepen, or maintain trance.
- Using pauses to create expectancy or unconscious creativity.
- Stretching out words to emphasise their meaning: "yeeeeees".
- Emphasising particular words to change the implication of a sentence (see Chapter 4).
- Using unclear pronunciation or unusual emphasis to create ambiguity.

New hypnotherapists might consider taking some acting or singing lessons to learn how to free their voice and discover what it can do.

Role-playing/miming

When using metaphors or analogies, Brooks not only tells the story; he enacts it. He steps into the role of a figure, character or object in the story, making it livelier. He thereby draws the client's attention, appeals to the unconscious (more childlike) mind and invites the client to engage in the story. In the Spider Phobia session, he does this towards the end where he creates a story/game in which the client is playing with the imaginary spider. It is almost as if he is talking to a child and engaging that child in play. In fact, he is talking to the client's inner child, allowing her to have a positive and joyful experience with a spider.

General movement and gesturing

Watching Brooks work with a client, you can see he uses a lot of body language. Even when the client has his or her eyes closed and cannot see him, he will use gestures, facial expressions, movements etc. As a former singer and performer, he feels free to use his body to express himself. On the one hand, body language is used specifically for analogue marking. On the other, Brooks uses it to be congruent, i.e. his body moves with his voice. When he talks about a cloud up there, he also looks and points up. He is convinced that when his movements match his words, he will sound more congruent. Brooks makes sure his gestures have the same rhythm and energy as his words; this means that the client will unconsciously pick up on this congruence and be more likely to follow his suggestions.

Chapter 7: Trance

Trance as an everyday experience

Trance is a natural experience that frequently happens in everyday life. Whenever someone is focused on something rather than switching his awareness between various objects or phenomena, he is in a certain trance. This can happen when someone reads a book, watches a movie, performs a task or is engaged in a conversation. These are all examples of an externally-oriented trance: the person is focused on or involved in something from the outside world. There is a strong interaction between the object of their focus and their own internal world of thoughts and feelings. If, however, someone drifts off or starts daydreaming, he detaches from the external world and focuses on internal aspects like ideas, memories, fantasies etc. This is an internally-oriented trance. Both external and internal trances can happen spontaneously and are not usually recognised as trances by onlookers.

Therapeutic trance

In hypnotherapy, trance is deliberately induced for therapeutic intervention and problem-solving. It is goal-oriented and intended to free the client from a symptom, problem or difficulty and to reach personal goals. The trance allows the client to escape the limitations of the conscious mind and explore the potential of the unconscious. As Erickson stated (Erickson, Rossi, & Rossi, 1976):

> "Patients have problems because their conscious programming has too severely limited their capacities. The solution is to help them break through the limitations of their conscious attitudes to free their unconscious potential for problem-solving."

A hypnotherapeutic trance is usually an internally-oriented trance where the client focuses on his or her own thoughts, images, feelings etc. It can, however, start with an external focus, e.g. on a spot in the room (eyes open) and then shift to an internal focus on thoughts and feelings (eyes closed). An interesting case is a person in a deep trance who is hallucinating. The person hallucinating has his or her eyes open and is focused on something external that is not really there. Actually, he or she is focusing on an internal image, which he or she believes to exist in external reality.

Trance as interpersonal experience

A hypnotherapeutic trance is different from an everyday spontaneous trance in that it involves another person. It is the hypnotherapist that induces or elicits the state of trance. In traditional hypnosis, this is done in an authoritarian way in that the hypnotist tells the client, in a direct way, to go into trance. It is the hypnotist's suggestion that 'leads' the client to go into trance. This is very useful in dental or medical hypnosis to induce trance for relaxation or anaesthesia. In psychotherapy, however, is it usually better to elicit the client's natural trance-ability. Here, trance is part of a therapeutic change process. Brooks might use an induction ritual and some vague suggestions initially, to get the induction process started, but then he 'follows' and ratifies the client's natural trance behaviour. He observes subtle trance phenomena that happen spontaneously and reinforces them. The state of trance helps the client to let go of rational and conscious control in favour of unconscious responses. With the exception of self-hypnosis, hypnotic trance is an interpersonal experience. As Rossi describes (Erickson, Rossi, & Rossi, 1976):

> "Trance is a special state that intensifies the therapeutic relationship and focuses the client's attention on a few inner realities."

Brooks is an expert in creating that special relationship. Upon the first contact, he himself enters an externally-oriented trance of focus, warmth, humour and trust. This creates an intense rapport with the client that helps him or her to experience trance, to allow unconscious processes to happen and to explore unconscious resources and solutions.

Trance as a gateway to the unconscious

A trance is a state where conscious control is decreased, and unconscious expression is increased. Brooks strongly believes that problem solution occurs by allowing the unconscious mind to let things happen automatically. The experience of trance frees the unconscious mind from conscious influence and allows it to express itself. Sometimes it is enough to observe and encourage this unconscious process, allowing the unconscious to explore, review and restructure the associational network and thereby solve the problem. Ernest Rossi's technique of Mirroring Hands (Hill & Rossi, 2017) (Rossi & Cheek, 1988) is a good example of this minimal intervention process.

Often, it is useful or necessary to help the unconscious along, with artfully vague suggestions, therapeutic rituals (techniques) or metaphors. In trance, the unconscious can easily pick up our vague suggestions and translate them to concrete images, feelings and actions. It can express unconscious feelings, needs and desires and develop creative ideas, possibilities and solutions. Unconscious activity can be experienced by the client in the form of feelings, sensations, automatic movements and internal images. It can be observed by the hypnotherapist in the form of visible cues like involuntary movements, pupil dilation, muscle relaxation, tears etc. Sometimes the unconscious expresses itself to the hypnotherapist but not to the client, by making sure a response can be seen but not felt. As one of my (JvB) clients once said, "I heard you say 'thank you' several times, but I had no idea what you were thanking me for". I was, in fact, thanking her unconscious mind for the very subtle ideomotor finger movements that she did not feel. Brooks talks about a confidential therapeutic encounter between the patient's unconscious and the therapist. In a light trance, the client's conscious mind usually observes the unconscious process from a distance and can report what happens. In a deep trance the conscious mind can totally drift off or become passive, and the entire unconscious process might happen unnoticed. A third possibility is that the client witnessing the trance consciously experiences what happens, but has amnesia about what happened after the session is over.

Trance and reality

Like Erickson, Brooks considers trance to be a state with an altered relationship to reality. The development of trance usually begins by limiting the number of referents of external reality. The client might focus on a spot in the room or on the therapist's eyes. He or she might receive the suggestion to be aware only of the feeling in his or her hands, or to restrict listening to the hypnotherapist's voice. While trance develops, irrelevant sensory triggers become blocked out, leaving the client aware only of the stimuli that are part of the hypnotic situation. As well as this reduction of external stimuli, trance involves a shift from external reality to internal reality. When the client closes his or her eyes, awareness changes from external objects and events to internal images and feelings. Even external sounds —except the hypnotherapist's voice— can fade away and make room for internal sounds, voices, music etc. A similar thing happens when a person falls asleep when, with the exception of important or unusual sounds, external reality is replaced by the internal reality of dreams. The shift from external to internal is also a shift from conscious to unconscious control. The deeper the trance a person is in, the more the unconscious mind determines his or her functioning, including internal images, feelings, sensations and movements. While the conscious mind has a limited number of referents in terms of perceptions, thoughts, feelings and actions, the unconscious has a huge number of referents, based on a lifetime of experiences and an open imagination. While trance reduces the number of conscious external referents, it increases the number of unconscious internal referents. Unconscious referents allow the client to find new behaviours, meanings, responses and feelings, which can be explored, activated and then integrated in external reality. As Erickson wrote (Erickson, Rossi, & Rossi, 1976):

> "We hypothesise that in everyday life consciousness is in a continual state of flux between the general reality orientation and the momentary micro-dynamics of trance.... The well-trained hypnotherapist is one who is acutely aware of these dynamics and their behavioural manifestations. Trance experience and hypnotherapy are simply the extension and utilisation of these normal psychodynamic processes."

In the Spider Phobia session, the client lives in an external reality where both the image of spiders and the places they might be, play a major role. For most people, spiders are irrelevant referents, which have no influence on their relationship with reality. For this client, spiders 'determine' her relationship with the external world. Brooks leads her into trance by reducing her external referents to the sensation in her arm, the image of her ring and the sound of his voice. The audience, the world and all the spiders in it start to disappear. She then orients herself to the internal reality of herself on a beach where anything is possible and where she can start to change her relationship with the 'concept spider' in a safe and creative way. Towards the end of the session, this new relationship is transferred to the external world, beginning with the building where the session takes place, and into her future through posthypnotic suggestions.

Trance as a state of suggestibility

When a client is in trance, he or she is more open to suggestion. The critical conscious mind is depotentiated so suggestions can enter the unconscious mind more easily. Obviously, there are two sides to this. In an uncritical state, not only can positive, constructive, and suitable suggestions flow in, but negative, destructive, or unsuitable ones as well. This is actually happening all the time in daily life. It is especially true of children, whose critical minds have not fully developed, leaving them vulnerable to all kinds of suggestions, both positive and negative. But adults too can be in a state of openness or trance in various situations and are therefore also open to suggestions both good and bad. Some people have a strong external reference, which means they tend to believe what others say, no matter what state they are in. As a hypnotherapist, you have the best intentions regarding your client and provide positive and helpful suggestions; the problem is you don't always know if a suggestion will be helpful or suitable. This is particularly true at the beginning of the therapeutic process, when you don't yet know your client's needs, patterns, thinking style or beliefs. In Ericksonian hypnotherapy, there are a couple of ways to deal with this. First, be artfully vague, pacing and leading your client, avoiding any specific mismatches. The client will unconsciously turn your vague words into concrete images, feelings and actions. Secondly, observe your client's nonverbal responses to whatever you say. The client might gently nod when you say something that fits, or shake his or her head when you say something that doesn't. Look for any cues that let you know if your words resonate with the client or not. More important than saying the right things is noticing the response to what you say and utilising that response. When I (JvB) see nonverbal disagreement to what I say, I simply add "or maybe something else..." and watch for the response to that. Brooks sometimes uses a meta-suggestion —a suggestion about suggestions— for this purpose. For example, he might say the client can translate all his words into his or her own words or that his suggestions will only work if they support the client's health and wellbeing. These meta-suggestions empower the client to use suggestions selectively and flexibly and provide another way to avoid the incorporation of unsuitable suggestions. One further consideration is that a person's unconscious mind doesn't follow every suggestion unconditionally. Experiments have shown that, even in deep trance, people do not do things that are in conflict with their core values and ethical boundaries.

Trance induction

Brooks sometimes induces trance as part of a seemingly casual conversation. He might talk about the client's everyday life, including work, family or hobbies. Very often people show subtle signs of trance when talking about something of interest. More specifically, Brooks might ask about previous trance experiences or the client's ideas on hypnosis. He or she then needs to (re)create certain aspects of trance to answer the question. As soon as the client starts to show signs of trance, Brooks will utilise these for further induction and deepening. Trance induction in Ericksonian hypnotherapy is not a standardised procedure. It is about utilising the client's behaviour, responses, experiences, thinking style and beliefs. If a client believes that hypnotherapy must require an induction ritual, Brooks will use one simply to convince the client's conscious mind that hypnosis is done. He chooses from a large number of available induction rituals —fixation, fascination, visualisation, arm levitation, catalepsy, confusion, self-talk etc. — to match and utilise the client's verbal or nonverbal expressions. If the client raises an arm repeatedly while talking, or uses words like 'up', 'higher' or 'lifting', an arm levitation induction might be appropriate. I (JvB) often use the fascination induction when a client looks (stares) at me expectantly, waiting for hypnosis to begin. Trance can be induced indirectly by using embedded suggestions, metaphor or by talking about someone else going into trance. The latter is known as Erickson's 'my friend John' technique (Erickson & Rossi, 1980a). In any case, the principle of trance induction is utilisation. Brooks constantly looks for signs of pupil dilation, changes in blinking or breathing, stillness etc. Utilising these signals may involve:

- mentioning cues, e.g. "your eyes are blinking".
- ratifying cues, e.g. by saying "yes", "okay", "that's right" when they occur.
- mirroring cues, e.g. blinking with your own eyelids in the same rhythm.
- coinciding cues with deepening suggestions, e.g. saying "deeper" with every blink.

Induction can also be completely nonverbal. Milton Erickson was famous for his handshake induction in which he would shake the client's hand and release it in a slow and confusing way. I (JvB) have sometimes induced trance simply by synchronising my blinking with that of the client, first pacing his or her blinking and then leading it.

A special induction using verbal and nonverbal elements developed by Brooks is called 'insertive eye contact'. Here he uses analogue marking, directing his gaze and voice to one side of the face or the other, depending on whether he is addressing the conscious or unconscious mind. All of this may sound a bit overwhelming if you are a new or inexperienced therapist. Not to worry; if the concept of utilisation is unfamiliar, just pick any induction technique and deliver it with all your heart. If it doesn't seem to work (i.e. if the client does not show signs of trance), gently switch to another technique; even Milton Erickson did not always get people into trance immediately. His secret was to be flexible and utilise whatever the client gave him, moment by moment. Every response, whether compliant or resistant, gave him valuable information for the next step. He was very confident that he would get there and that, sooner or later, people would go into trance. Brooks has that same high level of confidence; that certainty that he will get there, that the client will develop a certain level of trance and that he or she will solve the problem. He fully accepts everything the client says or does and utilises it. Once you understand this idea and know how to use it, trance induction becomes fairly easy. The conscious mind will give up resisting because there is nothing left to resist, not when every behaviour is interpreted as cooperation. Trance will develop as a natural state for relaxing, recovering, healing and growth. The unconscious mind is free to express its wisdom and power.

In the Spider Phobia session, Brooks uses a combination of two induction techniques:

- Fixation: he has the client fixate her gaze on the ring on her finger.
- Catalepsy: he immobilises her right arm by lifting it and then gently pushing it up and down and sideways in a confusing manner.

Apart from these rituals, he observes and utilises her responses to maintain and deepen trance at various points in the session.

Trance phenomena

Classical phenomena of hypnotic trance are catalepsy, anaesthesia, amnesia, hallucination, ideomotor signalling and automatic writing. These phenomena can occur spontaneously or as a result of suggestion, typically when the person is in deep trance. There are, however, many phenomena that happen in a light trance or that are signs of trance beginning:

- a sense of relaxation, comfort or heaviness.
- stillness/immobility of the body.
- smoothing out of facial muscles.
- changes in breathing, blinking and swallowing.
- changes in skin colour.
- increased pupil dilation.
- illusions of body size/shape.
- eye closure or staring.
- increased imagery.
- hypermnesia (increased memory).
- time distortion.
- time regression or progression.
- dissociation.
- things happening all by themselves.

Observing these phenomena is an important skill, for they can all be utilised to induce or deepen trance. Even the slightest signal of trance can be observed and then reinforced by suggestion. It is as if you are saying to the unconscious, "I see what you are doing; keep on doing that and do more of it". Some phenomena, like pupil size, always change in one direction (dilation) when the client goes into trance. Other phenomena, like the frequency of blinking or breathing, can change in both directions. For these, it is important to know the client's baseline: the state of that phenomenon in his or her normal waking state. Ideomotor responses can happen spontaneously in the form of finger movements, head nods or other kinds of involuntary movement. Alternatively, they can be set up for specific communication between the unconscious and the hypnotherapist. A typical technique is to choose a certain finger for a yes-response and another one for a no-response. Then to ask the unconscious various yes/no questions about the problem or its solution. Another is automatic writing or automatic drawing. This is a difficult trance phenomenon for a client to experience, and usually requires some practice, but it allows for more flexible communication with the unconscious.

The experience of trance is highly individual, and people vary a lot in their capacity to experience certain phenomena. Some people visualise easily; when they think about something, they will see images in their mind, remembered or fantasised. They can review past experiences, imagine future possibilities or perform any other visual task. Other people more readily experience physical sensations and movement. When they think about something, they might feel warm or cold, heavy or light, sensitive or numb. In trance, they often exhibit involuntary movement of their fingers, arms, head or other parts of the body. Many hypnotherapists are highly skilled in guided visualisation but not so much in guided kinaesthetic/motor experience. Utilisation also means using the channel that is most developed or more prominent with respect to the problem. Any trance phenomenon, and the sensory experience that goes with it can be utilised for the client's benefit.

Brooks usually looks for spontaneous phenomena and capitalises on them. Alternatively, he might suggest various trance phenomena to find out what works best. If the client 'fails' to experience a certain phenomenon, this is never a problem. In Ericksonian hypnotherapy, every response is considered an unconscious choice. As such, there is no failure; the client is always doing well. Brooks continuously validates the unconscious, no matter what it does, and invites it to further express itself. In the Spider Phobia session, he frequently says to the client "...doing very, very well." The client will get the feeling of being truly understood and appreciated.

Trance phenomena are important convincers. They prove to the client that something unusual is happening, something out of their rational and conscious control. It convinces them that they are really in hypnosis. This, in turn, proves that they will get better. Of course, this is not necessarily true, but when the client believes it, it is more likely to become true.

A trance phenomenon can also be a metaphor for the problem, the solution, or any aspect of the client's life. A cataleptic arm can represent a problem state of rigidity or being stuck; releasing the catalepsy then means becoming more flexible or active in life. For someone who experiences him or herself as weak, a cataleptic arm can represent firmness or power. I (JvB) often use catalepsy for smoking cessation as a metaphor for being unable to lift a cigarette. I sometimes add the posthypnotic suggestion of '*the arm getting this way, whenever necessary*'[43].

In the Spider Phobia session, arm catalepsy is induced at the beginning of the session as a part of trance induction. At the end, the rigid arm serves as proof of Brooks' influence on the client (utilising her external reference) and the power of her own unconscious mind. Along the way, he redefines her 'inability' to move her arm, transforming it into the 'ability' to make her arm rigid. Finally, Brooks links her ability to make her arm rigid to her ability to overcome her fear and feel comfortable with spiders. This catalepsy and its release is also a metaphor for her problem (a lifetime of rigidly holding on to a fear and the inability to let it go) and its solution (releasing herself from the fear). Another trance phenomenon, the trembling of her eyelids, is defined as proof of her being a good hypnotic subject and as a way of helping her to solve her problem. But the main trance phenomenon in this session is dissociation, a double VK (visual-kinaesthetic) dissociation. The client looks at herself looking at herself. The phenomenon of imagery is used increasingly throughout the session. The client visualises herself on the beach; she visualises clouds, words and spiders in the clouds etc. Amnesia for certain suggestions is created by using amnesia gaps

[43] A vague suggestion for the arm to become rigid whenever the urge to smoke arises.

(saying the same words before and after the suggestion) and by switching to irrelevant topics.

Trance depth

Brooks has no fixed ideas about the depth of trance required for certain phenomena or changes to happen. He induces a level of trance that is possible as well as safe for a client and necessary for the problem to be solved. A client can go in and out of trance many times and the trance depth can vary throughout the session. Trance can also be partial, with respect to the sensory systems. A client can be internally oriented (in trance) in one sensory system while externally oriented in another. Brooks uses this phenomenon to stay in verbal contact with the client during trance. The client can experience imagery and sensations (visually and kinaesthetically in trance) while being able to talk about it (auditory, out of trance). Trance induction can also be fractionated, meaning the client is led in and then out of trance several times, going deeper with each repeat. In Ericksonian hypnotherapy, hypnotisability is not considered a fixed trait of a client as it is in traditional hypnosis. Whether or not a client goes into trance and the trance depth he or she achieves depends on previous trance experience, the hypnotherapist's verbal and nonverbal skills, the interpersonal relationship between client and therapist and the amount of time spent developing it. Ernest Rossi wrote about trance (Erickson & Rossi, 1981):

> "The concept of trance depth is highly relative. Erickson likes to point out that a trance can be both deep and light at the same time. It can be deep in the sense that a person is so absorbed that he or she does not notice irrelevant stimuli like the traffic outside or a surgical tray dropped a few feet away. The trance is light in the sense that important and relevant stimuli like the therapist's voice are easily received."

Trance, metaphor, and tasking

Hypnotic trance is an important aspect of Ericksonian hypnotherapy. Trance is the state where the unconscious is more accessible, more active and free to express itself. The state of trance makes therapeutic suggestions more effective, or as Brooks puts it, "trance is an adhesive; it makes suggestions stick." Nevertheless, it is not always necessary or appropriate to use trance. For example, when a client needs to stay alert for an important phone call or when a client's condition, e.g. psychosis, is a contraindication to trance induction.

As well as hypnotic trance, Brooks utilises two other Ericksonian pathways: metaphor and tasking. These can be used in combination with trance or as separate interventions. Sometimes Brooks' only intervention is giving a therapeutic task. The actual therapy is the performance of the task. Other times he spends an entire session creating metaphors and analogies that reflect the client's problem and its solution. Even a task can be given in the form of a metaphor. In most sessions, especially in teaching demonstrations, Brooks uses all three pathways: trance, metaphor and tasking. The Spider Phobia session begins with a few analogies, is followed by an extensive trance experience that contains a metaphor and ends with a task.

Learning trance induction

In many courses on hypnosis and hypnotherapy trance induction is taught in the form of one or more techniques. In Ericksonian hypnosis, trance induction is about something different. It begins with building rapport and gaining your client's trust. Only then can a client enter and develop his own natural and individual process of trance. The role of the hypnotherapist is to observe the signals of beginning trance and encourage and utilise them. Trance develops from within and in full accordance with the client's pace, needs and hypnotic style. For some people, observation and stimulation of their natural tendency to go into trance is enough. Others may need a little more help in the form of seeding ideas about possible trance phenomena, confusing the conscious mind or creating a double bind to make trance inevitable. It is, therefore, a good idea to learn about all these things. Although Ericksonian trance induction is never a predefined ritual, it is valuable to learn and master some of the formal rituals like eye fixation, fascination, visualisation and hand levitation. If a client has a fixed idea about hypnosis and expects a ritual, a predefined ritual might be required. Ultimately, the ability to lead people into trance effectively is about developing your own hypnotic personality. Then your mere presence will induce trance in your clients. Brooks reached this level many years ago.

Chapter 8: Phobias

The client in the session described in this book has a fear of spiders; this is also known as arachnophobia. It is a one of the most common specific phobias that people can develop for objects, animals or situations. People with a specific phobia experience intense and immediate fear when they are confronted with the object or situation concerned. They usually know that their fear is irrational but have no control over their emotional and behavioural reaction. They tend to avoid places, situations or people that could trigger their fear.

Although specific phobias often have their roots in childhood, as a result of experiencing or witnessing traumatic events, they can also develop later in life. An explanation of phobic responses is given by Joseph Ledoux in his book 'The Emotional Brain' (Ledoux, 1996). He explains how the emotional response to a certain stimulus occurs via two different channels: the low road —via the sensory thalamus and the amygdala— and the high road, via the sensory thalamus, the cortex and the amygdala. The low road performs a fast and crude appraisal of a stimulus, based on information from the implicit memory systems. The high road performs a slow, detailed and rational appraisal of the stimulus, based on information in the explicit memory systems.

Children can have all kinds of irrational fears, which can be instinctive or learned. When they get older, they usually learn to think more rationally, to distinguish between real and unreal dangers and to overcome their unnecessary fears. The high road becomes stronger as the low road responses are controlled or extinguished. Normal experiences are stored as an integrated gestalt of sensory representations, physical feelings, emotions, and meaning, located in time and space and related to one's life story and identity. As Van der Kolk puts it: "...nontraumatic experiences are not registered in consciousness as separate sensory elements of the experience, but are automatically integrated into a coherent personal narrative." (Van der Kolk, McFarlane, & Weisaeth, 2007).

However, in the case of trauma, whether a victim or a witness, explicit memory formation is hindered by the reduced function of the hippocampus. The traumatic experience is stored as fragmented images, sounds and feelings, disconnected from time, place, or meaning. Van der Kolk further writes: "Traumatic memories are timeless and ego-alien." Any trigger reminding of the traumatic memory evokes the low-road emotional and behavioural response and the reality-oriented cognition of the high-road [44] is weak or absent.

[44] Which might, for example, tell he person "this is in the past", "this is harmless" or "it's not my fault".

Hypnotherapy allows people to heal traumatic memories and/or replace them with positive ones. The Spider phobia session described in this book is an example of the latter, the creation of a positive experience with a spider. Subtle indirect suggestions, however, are also used to resolve her traumatic memories. Healing trauma also involves changing limiting beliefs that have developed as a result of traumatic experiences.

Most people with arachnophobia do not consciously believe that spiders are dangerous. They do, however, build various beliefs around their phobia. Someone with a spider phobia might develop anticipatory fear based on the belief "when I see a spider, I'll panic". In the course of time, other beliefs arise about people ("they think I am crazy"), places ("I have to avoid all places where there might be spiders"), time ("it will get worse or I'll never get over it") and identity ("I am a phobic"). They often arrange their life patterns and relationships around their phobia. After several years of living with a phobia, the problem is a complexity of unresolved traumatic memories, conditioned responses and various limiting beliefs.

Traditionally phobias were treated with Behavioural Therapy using systematic desensitisation. Nowadays, a number of approaches are available such as CBT, EMDR, NLP and classical hypnosis. All of these approaches can work, but their limitation is that they use more or less the same procedure for any client. Each phobia is different, however, and one person's spider phobia is not exactly like someone else's. In Ericksonian hypnotherapy, we tailor the session to each individual client utilising their phobic responses, life patterns, beliefs, thinking style and personality. This allows the client to resolve his or her fear safely, effectively and in full accordance with his or her needs, values, and boundaries.

The client in the session described in this book seems to have developed her spider phobia as a result of watching her mother panic. She has an intense fear response when she sees a spider or something she thinks is a spider. Behavioural aspects of the problem are checking cupboards, beds, sofas etc. for possible spiders before cleaning or using them. She has had the kinaesthetic hallucination of spiders crawling up her legs when she knew or suspected them to be in the room. Just thinking about a spider is enough for her to feel the fear. Her problem seems to have a strong social aspect. She developed it as a child, watching her mother panic and now she is starting to transfer her fear to her daughter. The client describes a few of the panic attacks she has experienced when confronted with spiders and how her phobia influences her daily activities. With respect to her problem, she seems to have an external reference (her mother has sent her to therapy) and an external locus of control (she does not believe she can solve it herself). She hints at a possible limiting belief that her problem is hereditary. All of these aspects of her problem and her personality are utilised by Brooks to create a highly personalised hypnotherapy session.

PART TWO

Spider Phobia Session Verbatim and Analysis

Synopsis

The Spider Phobia session described is a demonstration in front of an audience. Brooks has only met the client briefly before the session and does not know her in any other way. The client has a severe spider phobia and has requested Brooks' help to get over it. Brooks starts by helping her feel comfortable on the stage by giving compliments and by using humour. He gathers some information about her problem, he normalises her fear and defines it as easy to solve. Brooks establishes a frame of success by referring to previous effective treatment of similar problems. Trance induction is performed with a combination of arm catalepsy, eye fixation and imagination. The client's favourite place is also utilised as a context for the therapeutic intervention that follows. This intervention consists of an extended visualisation in which Brooks leads the client through the experience and resolution of her problem. The main techniques used are those of double dissociation and hypnotic desensitisation. Brooks enables her to gradually look at spiders while feeling comfortable and in control. Spiders are indirectly reframed from 'dangerous creatures' to 'harmless friends'.

Brooks subtly and indirectly hands over the role of therapist to the client. At the end of the session, the client has become the therapist, and she is now a friend of the spider; a role reversal of the original problem situation and a metaphor for the client being her own therapist. The solution is integrated at the level of her identity and transferred to the external world, her family network and her future. Immediately after the session, the client is asked to explore the corridors of the hospital to find spiders and test her response. This she does with enthusiasm, successfully making lots of new 'spider friends' and allowing them to crawl onto her hands without any recurrence of her previous fear.

NLP practitioners will recognise the double dissociation phobia technique as developed by Richard Bandler (Bandler, 1985). Behavioural and cognitive behavioural therapists will note that a desensitisation process is used. Brooks' demonstration, however, differs from the standard NLP technique and from the behavioural desensitisation technique in a number of ways:

- A state of hypnotic trance is used. It is induced at the beginning, maintained throughout the session and ratified at the end.
- Brooks utilises the client's favourite place of relaxation as a context for the dissociation rather than the standard NLP metaphor of a

movie theatre. Clouds in the sky are utilised as a projection screen for therapeutic imagery.

- Hypnotic (imaginal) desensitisation is used rather than in vivo desensitisation. As such, the process is under the therapist's control, and complete problem resolution occurs within the session. Desensitisation happens in two successive modalities, first the digital (words) and then the visual (images) modality.
- Brooks uses vague language, indirect suggestion, implication, metaphor and analogy rather than direct suggestion or instructions.
- Brooks induces and utilises trance phenomena like eye fluttering and catalepsy to ratify the work.
- The double dissociation and hypnotic desensitisation are not chosen beforehand as a standard technique to cure a phobia. It develops during the session in response to the client's communication.
- Throughout the session, Brooks demonstrates the main principles of his work: observation-utilisation. He carefully listens to her words, observes her minimal cues, and utilises her communication to help her solve the problem.

Conventions in this transcript

Underlined: embedding linguistic structure: the wrapping of the actual suggestion.

I'd like you to *learn something else.*

Italics: direct or embedded suggestion for the unconscious mind [45].

I'd like you to *learn something else.*

Italics bold: key suggestions for problem resolution and self-esteem.

feel perfectly okay in the future

SMALL CAPITALS: words that create a link between one idea or experience and another.

Keep looking at that ring AS *you are on the beach.*

Open your eyes AND see if *you can feel comfortable.*

---

[45] Or a suggestion that involves the conscious and the unconscious mind. Behavioural instructions for the conscious mind are not in italics.

He is *feeling much more comfortable* - BECAUSE *he can trust her.*

Symbol ⊇ : presupposition

It is <u>another</u> learn-problem ⊇ there are more learn-problems

means: It is <u>another</u> learn-problem – presupposes - there are more learn-problems

Symbol ⊃ : implication

Hear the sound of my voice ⊃ don't hear the words

means: Hear the sound of my voice - implies - don't hear the words

(5 sec.): a 5-second pause between words

...: a pause less than 5 seconds between words

Stretched out words: indicated by repeated letters

Veeery deeply relaaaxed

Superscripts used to indicate forms of embedded suggestion:

DM = Discourse Marker
SA = Sentence Adverb
MO = Modal Operator
ER = Explicit Request
A = Announcement
TF = Verb of thinking and feeling
FV = Factive Verb
Q = Quote
TQ = Tag Question
LS = Linguistic Softener
QA = Qualifying Adjective
NP= Noun Phrase
EQ = Embedded Question
DA = Degree Adverb
TA = Time Adverb
PA = Place Adverb

Verbatim

Below, you will find a verbatim transcript of the entire Spider Phobia session. After every couple of minutes, there is a descriptive interpretation of what happened, the choices Brooks has made and their meaning. This is then followed by a list of language patterns and techniques in the piece. For readability purposes, only the main language patterns are listed. Frequently occurring vague words like 'thing', 'thought', 'feeling', 'to think', 'to be aware', 'to do' etc. are not listed. As described in Chapter 4, every nominalisation presupposes the thing it describes to exist. The word 'change' presupposes 'change' to exist. These simple presuppositions will not be listed unless they are especially relevant. Suggestions are listed as embedded whenever they are wrapped up in certain words or phrases as described in part I of this book. Others are listed as direct suggestions. The distinction between indirect (embedded) and direct suggestions is not always clear-cut, however. Direct suggestions, although not embedded at sentence-level, can still be embedded in the larger linguistic structure and vice versa, indirect suggestions might come across as direct because of the way they are pronounced. Some suggestions are overt instructions for the client's conscious mind whereas others are covert messages for her unconscious mind. Also, the difference between suggestions and statements is not always obvious because, in hypnotherapy, statements often act as suggestions. Although the embedding structure serves as wrapping material for the actual suggestion, it may contain suggestions on its own. Questions can be requests for information from the conscious or unconscious mind, and they may contain embedded suggestions. Questions always hold certain implications, and they are listed as such. Brooks' communication is a continuous flow of interwoven and interacting suggestions (direct and indirect), statements, questions and implications, that is strongly influenced by body language and intonation. Identifying and describing the individual components of his communication with a client can never be complete, nor can it do justice to the holistic nature of the hypnotic encounter. It is, however, necessary for educational purposes.

Start of the session

Brooks gives the microphone to the client and instructs her to put it on. The client is looking at the audience. She seems to be a little nervous.

Brooks: (while she puts on the microphone) So we can hear you scream.

> Brooks uses humour here to make the client feel comfortable. He also permits her, indirectly, to speak up, by taking it to the extreme (to scream). When Brooks is working with a client, a joke is never just a joke.

Client: (smiling, looking at the audience, then looking at Brooks) Is that okay?

Brooks: Yes. Well, hmm, take a few moments to *get used to this mob* out here. *They are quite harmless*, they haven't got wings.

> Let's have a look at these two sentences. Therapy has already started. Brooks uses an implied link, suggesting that 'taking a few moments' causes 'getting used to them'. He also suggests that the crowd is harmless by saying they are *quite harmless.* Quite harmless is easier to believe than harmless, which would mean entirely harmless. At the same time, the qualifying adverb *quite* turns harmless into a presupposition; *quite harmless* presupposes *harmless.* The conscious mind is tied up with the question of how harmless *quite harmless* is, while the unconscious mind can pick up the word *harmless.* Brooks then provides 'proof' of the crowd being harmless by linking harmlessness to not having wings. Obviously, this is not real proof, but it might just make it a little easier to believe. While the conscious mind is entertained by the humour of it, the unconscious can pick up the implied message "they are harmless". The idea of harmlessness has been seeded here and will be applied to spiders later in the session.
>
> Embedded suggestions:
>
> - Well[DM], hmm, take a few moments[TA] to *get used to this mob* out here[PA].
>
> Implied cause-effect link:
>
> - *They are quite harmless* - (BECAUSE) they haven't got wings.

Vague language:

- Vague verb: get used to
- Vague adjective: harmless
- Unspecified person: we, this mob, they
- Unspecified time: a few moments

Presuppositions:

- Qualifying adverb:
  quite harmless ⊇ harmless

Various techniques:

- Humour: so we can hear you scream, this mob, they haven't got wings
- Analogy: harmless mob stands for harmless spiders

Client: (Smiling and looking at Brooks) They have got legs though.

Brooks: They have got legs (laughs), yeeeess. Not very long ones ... and usually only two each.

The client does not immediately accept the harmlessness of the audience and argues that people have legs (like spiders). As such, she indirectly lets Brooks know that her fear of spiders might be related to them having legs. Brooks acknowledges her words by repeating them and then reframing them by saying that the people's legs are not long and there are only two. This is a kind of response often used by Brooks: acknowledging the problem and then limiting it (only two legs). The phrase 'usually only two' makes it funny and confusing, because people, by definition, have no more than two legs. To process this sentence, the client has to think (unconsciously) of beings with more than two legs. In the context of the session, she will probably think of spiders, and a subtle link is created between (harmless) people and spiders.

Embedded statements:

- Usually[SA] only two each.

Vague language:

- Unspecified person: they
- Unspecified object: ones, two

Presuppositions:

- Qualifying adverb:
  not very long ones ⊇ not long ones

Various techniques:

- Reframing: not very long ones.
- Humour: usually only two each.

Brooks: Okay, so get ... take a while to *get used to the feeling of being up here.* It's quite an unusual thing to be up here in front of people, I'm sure. Have you ever been in a situation like this before?

Here, Brooks normalises the client's experience of nervousness. First, he does so implicitly 'take a while to get used to'…and then explicitly 'it's quite an unusual thing'. Brooks does this a lot, suggesting something both implicitly and explicitly. It's a way of repeating the same message in different forms. The suggestion 'take a while to get used to...' not only normalises, it also tells her that she *will* get used to it. Brooks then frames the situation as unusual with a general remark, 'it's quite an unusual thing...', not directly referring to her. Then he makes it personal by asking her if she has experienced it before. This is another way of repeating a message, first deliver it generally, then personally. Brooks probably expects her to say no, but he would utilise any answer she might give.

Embedded suggestions:

- Okay[DM] so[DM] get.. take a while[TA] *to get used to the feeling of being up here.*

Embedded statements:

- It's quite an unusual thing to be up here in front of people, I'm sure[FV].

Vague language:

- Nominalisation: situation
- Unspecified person: people
- Unspecified time: a while
- Unspecified object/event: thing
- No personal pronoun (infinitive): It's quite an unusual thing to be up here.
- Mind reading: It's quite an unusual thing to be up here…

Presuppositions:

- Qualifying adverb:
  quite an unusual thing $\supseteq$ an unusual thing

Various techniques:

- Normalisation: it's quite an unusual thing to be up here

Client: (Shaking her head, smiling) No.

Brooks: Okay. So, just take a moment to *get used to it.* WHILE *you are doing that* (rotating his hands backwards), I would like you to, kind of collect your thoughts ... AND think about ... this ... this problem you've got.

> Brooks here repeats the suggestion of getting used to the audience. He then indirectly suggests she should think about her problem. Using dependent (while) and adjunctive (and) suggestions, he connects 'getting used to it' to 'collecting her thoughts' and to 'thinking about her problem'. From this moment on, she focuses on her inner experience and on Brooks. Initial rapport has been established, and she is responding. She is either looking at Brooks or staring into space (visualising); she only looks at the audience when Brooks asks her to do so.
>
> Embedded suggestions:
>
> - Okay[DM], so[DM] just[DA] take a moment[TA] to *get used to it.*
> - I would like you to[ER] kind of[LS] collect your thoughts.

Dependent/adjunctive suggestions:

- WHILE *you are doing that* - I would like you to, kind of collect your thoughts - AND think about this problem you've got.

Vague language:

- Nominalisation: problem
- Vague verb: get used to, collect
- Unspecified time: a moment
- Unspecified object/event: it, that

Presuppositions:

- Relative clause:
  this problem (that) you've got ⊇ you've got a problem

- Demonstrative determiner:
  <u>this</u> problem ⊇ there is a specific problem

Brooks: Hmm, first of all, how ... how were you recommended to come here?

With this request for factual information, Brooks distracts her conscious mind. This allows her unconscious to think about the problem, as he suggested before. How she was recommended is, in itself, an irrelevant question. Her answer will turn out to be relevant though since it reveals information about her thinking style, beliefs and family. Also, the word 'recommended' implies that this is something good.

Presuppositions:

- Ordinal numeral:
  <u>first</u> of all… ⊇ there will be more

- Question:
  <u>how</u> were you recommended to come here? ⊇ you were recommended to come here

Implications:

- how were you <u>recommended</u> to come here? ⊃ coming here is a good thing

Client: Hmm, through my mum (pointing behind her, over her right shoulder). She told me I should have something done about it, badly, because ... I've just got my ... I just had a little ... well she's 19 months, and she hmm, she ... when she sees me in the state, she gets in the state and uh ... of course it's not doing her any good.

> The client's thinking style seems to include both an external reference (my mother told me) and an external locus of control ('have something done about it' rather than 'do something about it') (Hall & Bodenhamer, 1997). Furthermore, her fear seems to include a systemic element; her mother points out the effect of her fear on her daughter. She labels her fear with a negative nominalisation (the state) and reveals a belief: "of course, that's not doing her any good." Brooks will utilise this belief of negative influence on her daughter later in a positive form.

Brooks: Hmm, hmm, can I tell you a story about that (turning to the audience). Somebody might know this story. Did you hear the story about the woman I went to see with a phobia about daddy-long-legs? Yeah.

> Overtly, Brooks is talking to the audience here, but covertly he is talking to her. By asking if someone knows the story, he increases her conscious curiosity and expectancy. A story about a daddy-long-legs phobia matches her indirect message that her fear has something to do with spiders' legs. Brooks' uses a rather flat, matter-of-fact voice tone here, matching her voice tone and hiding the significance of the story from her conscious mind.
>
> Vague language:
>
> - Nominalisation: story
> - Unspecified person: somebody, the woman
> - Unspecified object/event: that
>
> Presuppositions:
>
> - Relative clause:
>   the woman (<u>that</u>) I went to see ⊇ I went to see the woman
> - Demonstrative determiner:
>   <u>this</u> story ⊇ there is a specific story

Various techniques:

- Talking to others: talking to the audience
- Analogy: story about another client

Brooks: (turning to the client) I went to see a woman who had a daddy-long-legs phobia. I went to her house because she couldn't even leave the house at all (Client: Oh, yeah) you know. And ... and she said it was hereditary (looking at her).

Brooks here indirectly reduces the client's problem by talking about a woman with a similar but bigger problem (she couldn't 'even' leave the house 'at all'). This is a technique Brooks often uses, limiting the current problem to make it tangible and manageable.

Presuppositions:

- Relative clause:
  A woman <u>who</u> had a daddy-long-legs phobia ⊇ A woman had a daddy-long-legs phobia

- Qualifying adverb:
  She couldn't <u>even</u> leave the house <u>at all</u> ⊇ She couldn't leave the house

Implications:

- she couldn't even leave the house ⊃ her problem was worse than yours
- I went to her house ⊃ I am willing to make an effort to help someone
- <u>she said</u> it was hereditary ⊃ it was not hereditary

Client: Yeah?

Brooks: That's what she said to me. And I said: "Really?" and she said: "Yes, my mother had it." I said: "Really?" She said: "Yeah, and my daughter has got it, and now my son is getting it" and I said "Really?" So I said to her "Is this true?" And the little daughter said: "Yeah, I've got it." and I said to the little boy: "What happens there?" and he said: "Well every time one of these comes in the room, we all ... run under the stairs and play this game." (The client is smiling.) And I suddenly realised, in fact, that she'd been teaching it to the children. (The client nods, "yeah".) BUT it is not hereditary, it's impossible. (Client: "Yeah".) It cannot possibly be hereditary. It's not hereditary, BUT you can teach it (Client: "Mmm".) ... So congratulations on getting here now. (Client: smiles, plays with her fingers, "Yeah") ... SO THAT ***your family and your future family will be free from it***. (Client: "Mmm").

Brooks uses this story both to tackle her possible belief that her phobia is hereditary and to define it as a learned problem. By re-enacting a dialogue with the previous client, repeating the question "Really?" several times, he makes it clear that it was just the woman's idea that it was hereditary. The analogy also implies that Brooks has successfully worked with a similar client. As such, he demonstrates his competence and confidence, thereby increasing the client's trust. After telling her indirectly (by analogy), that the fear is not inherited, he then tells her directly ("it is not hereditary"). Then he tells her "you can teach it"; here, 'you' may refer to people in general or her specifically. She seems to apply it to herself. Before she could start feeling guilty about teaching the problem to her child, Brooks congratulates her. Her nonverbal response shows that the congratulation is a little confusing for her. Being congratulated implies she is doing something right (getting here now) rather than something wrong (teaching her child a problem). Her problem is now defined as 'something learned' and her behaviour as 'doing something about it so that her child can benefit'. The word 'congratulations' not only praises the client it also subtly transfers the responsibility for her presence from the mother to the client. Furthermore, her 'being here' is linked to the positive systemic effects on her family, implying a positive effect on herself (so that your family and your future family will be free from it).

Adjunctive suggestion:

- She'd been teaching it to the children - BUT it is not hereditary.
- It's not hereditary, BUT you can teach it.

Cause-effect link:

- Congratulations on getting here now - SO THAT *your family and your future family will be free from it.*

Embedded statements:

- I suddenly realised[FV] in fact[SA] that she'd been teaching it.

Direct statements:

- It's not hereditary, it's impossible.
- It cannot possibly be hereditary.

Vague language:

- Nominalisation: game
- Vague verb: to realise, to teach, to congratulate
- Vague adverb: really
- Vague adjective: free
- Unspecified person: we all, children, you, your (future) family
- Unspecified object/event: it, one of these

Presuppositions:

- Qualifying adverb:
  I suddenly realised $\supseteq$ I realised
  it cannot possibly be $\supseteq$ it cannot be

Implications:

- Really? Is this true? $\supset$ it is not true

Various techniques:

- Analogy: previous client with similar problem

Brooks: Okay, how long have you had this?

Brooks often starts a sentence with "Okay". With this word, he acknowledges what was said before or what happened before. The word is also a separator, a discourse marker, used to finish the previous communication and start a new one. At this point, he gathers more information about the problem. In Ericksonian hypnotherapy, information gathering, rapport building, induction and therapy happen simultaneously rather than sequentially.

Client: Ever since I was born.

Brooks: Since you were born?

Brooks waits a second before he responds and raises the pitch of his voice to sound surprised. He is playfully challenging her belief of having had the problem since birth.

Client: Well...(laughing)

The client immediately realises what she said is not true. She might, however, feel embarrassed about this.

Brooks: Yeah. Very good memory (briefly reaches out to touch her).

Brooks reaches out to her with his hand and gives her a compliment. He does so while laughing with her. In this way, she doesn't need to feel embarrassed and she can laugh about her belief of having the problem since birth. The compliment of her having a good memory is also a possible suggestion to have a 'good memory' about the origin of her fear.

Vague language:

- Nominalisation: memory
- Ambiguity (homonym): memory

Presuppositions:

- Question:
  <u>how long</u> have you had this? ⊇ you have had this for a while

- Qualifying adverb:
  <u>very</u> good memory ⊇ good memory

Various techniques:

- Complimenting: very good memory
- Humour: very good memory
- Physical support: reaching out to her
- Challenging a belief: since you were born?

Client: So, when my mum used to see one, she used to run, and of course I used to run with her (gesturing with her right arm to show the behaviour of running). (Brooks: "Yeah.") Client: I've been scared of it ever since she's been scared of it.

> The client now remembers and shares the experience that may have created her phobia of spiders. As a part of this memory, she shares a more specific belief: "…*of course* I used to run with her". It is another example of using her mother as an external reference. Her matter-of-fact way of saying, "I've been scared of it ever since she's been scared of it" seems to indicate that her mother's fear and her response (to run) is indeed the root of her problem. Brooks doesn't ask for more information at this point but continues to redefine the problem.

Brooks: Of course. So it is another learn-problem. (Client: "Yeah.")

> Brooks now directly connects the word 'problem' to the word 'learn'. He defines her problem as a 'learn-problem'. The client is very responsive. She alternates between looking at him (listening) and looking away (thinking) as he talks. She agrees verbally ("yeah") and nonverbally (subtly nodding).
>
> Embedded statement:
>
> - <u>So</u>[DM], it's another learn-problem.
>
> Vague language:
>
> - Nominalisation: learn-problem
> - Unspecified object/event: it
>
> Presuppositions:
>
> - Repetitive cue word:
>   it is <u>another</u> learn-problem ⊇ there are other learn-problems
>
> Techniques
>
> - Normalisation: of course

Brooks: The good thing about it being learned ... is, that ***it can be unlearned***... (Client: "Yeah"). Now if it was something which was organic (holding his hands close to his body), by that I mean, in medical terms, something which was like hereditary, like an illness that is passed down through the family ... (Client: "Hmm"), it's harder to work on, because it's like an organ in the body, that is affected in some way, BUT here ... it's a learned thing.

The client responds positively to the idea of the learning experience and, Brooks develops it further. He suggests that something that is learned can be unlearned. Of course, this is not an absolute fact, but Brooks presents it as such. Since the client has an external reference and the message is delivered indirectly, she will probably accept it as a fact. The frame of 'learning' is reinforced by contrasting her fear with an organic illness. The idea of 'something being hard to work on' is connected to an organic illness and by implication, disconnected from her fear so, again, Brooks is implying that her problem will be easy to solve. The word 'here' is ambiguous; it is a homophone of 'hear'. To her conscious mind, it means "here it is a learned thing". To her unconscious, it can also mean, "hear! It is a learned thing".

Embedded suggestions:

- The good thing[QA] about it, *it can be unlearned.*

Adjunctive suggestion:

- If it was something which was organic, it's harder to work on - BUT here it's a learned thing.

Vague language:

- Nominalisation: terms, illness, way
- Vague verb: learned, unlearned, passed down, work on
- Vague adjective: organic, medical
- Unspecified person: the family
- Unspecified place: here
- Unspecified object/event: thing, it, that, something, an organ
- Unspecified process: in some way
- Comparative deletion: harder
- No personal pronoun: it being learned

- Ambiguity (homophone): here/hear

Presuppositions:

- Noun-preposition:
  the good thing about it being learned is ⊇ there is something good about it being learned

- Counterfactual conditional clause:
  if it was something that was organic ⊇ it is not something organic

Various techniques:

- Reframing: 'hereditary problem' is reframed to 'learned thing'

Brooks: In the same way that, you know, you can ... you can *learn to recognise something* (analogue marking by stretching his hands forward), you know, it is just a question of learning, memory. So, BECAUSE it is a learned thing, we can *change it very easily.*

> Brooks further develops the idea of the problem being a learned thing by comparing it to other learning experiences and to memory. He already suggested that something learned can be unlearned. He now states directly what he suggested indirectly before: "because it is learned, we[46] can easily change it". The stepwise development of a positive belief is typical of Ericksonian hypnotherapy. As Erickson used to say: "you don't just throw something in, you work towards it". Brooks often works towards something by first implying something and then saying it explicitly. Obviously, his ideas are not absolute facts, but by stating them with a confident voice tone, posture and expression, the client can accept them and make them true. Ericksonian hypnotherapy is about using whatever idea will help to solve the problem and promote happiness, health, and well-being. Brooks utilises the client's external reference; she sees him as an expert and she will trust his judgment.

---

46 The client can interpret the word *we* as "*we hypnotherapists*" and feel taken care of, or as "*you and I*" and feel invited to cooperate and share responsibility. Either interpretation works in the right direction.

Embedded suggestions:

- You know[DM], you can[MO] *learn to recognise something.*

Cause-effect link:

- BECAUSE it is a learned thing - we can *change it very easily.*

Embedded statements:

- You know[DM], it is just a question of learning.

Vague language:

- Nominalisation: question, memory
- Vague verb: learn, recognise, change
- Unspecified person: we
- Unspecified object/event: something, it, thing
- Permissive: you can

Presuppositions

- Qualifying adverb:
  it is just a question of learning ⊇ it is a question of learning

  we can change it very easily ⊇ we can change it easily ⊇ we can change it

Brooks: Have you had any help with this?

Again, Brooks asks a closed (yes/no) question for factual information. The covert goal of this question is to distract her conscious mind from the suggestions he just gave her. Still, her answer can provide additional information that might be useful. Brooks uses the word 'help' here. This may seem an obvious word in any therapy session, but it is not. Using this word, he defines the session as 'help', tuning in to her obvious state of 'helplessness' with regards to spiders. With a less fearful client or someone with a more internal reference, he might have used a word like 'support' or 'guidance' or any description that would match the client's thinking style or expectancy. Later in the session, the word 'help' is utilised and reframed to 'her helping him to help her' and then to 'her helping herself'; this is a gradual process towards an internal locus of control.

Vague language:

- Nominalisation: help
- Unspecified object/event: this

Presuppositions:

- Simple presupposition:
  have you had any <u>help?</u> ⊇ help exists

Various techniques:

- Distraction: asking a question for facts to distract the conscious mind

Client: No, this is the first help I've had.

Her answer shows that she believes that help exists and that she sees this session as help.

Brooks: Okay (nodding). Now, you told me a little ... a few minutes ago, where I asked you, out there, about the problem, that ... you even got scars on your legs (pointing to her legs).

By nodding and saying okay, Brooks lets her know that it is okay that this is the first help she has received. He now distracts her conscious mind further by referring to the moments just before the session began. As such, he enhances amnesia for all the suggestions he has given her so far and gathers more information about the problem. Furthermore, he brings her attention to the concept of legs (hers or a spider's), which seems to be a relevant part of her fear. The word 'even' confirms the severity of the problem and it implies there are other serious aspects to it. Her story makes it clear that she has a big problem and Brooks acknowledges that implicitly.

Vague language:

- Nominalisation: problem
- Unspecified time: a few minutes ago

- Unspecified place: out there

Various techniques:

- Enhancing amnesia: referring to an earlier point in the session.

Client: Yeah, I've got scars on my legs (pointing to her legs) where I scratched myself because I think they're ... crawling up my legs.

> The client here shares a specific part of her problem, the kinaesthetic hallucination of a spider crawling up her legs and her scratching in response to it. Brooks will utilise the idea of spiders crawling up her body towards the end of the session and turn it into a positive experience.

Brooks: Uh-huh

Client: Uh once one episode was when there was one on the wall and I've gone out to find someone to get it out from there, and as I've come back down it's gone. And I thought it was on the carpet and I thought it was going up my legs and I scratched my legs. We've actually found it in the end, but uh until we found it I couldn't get back into the flat.

> The client tells the experience in a more or less dissociated way. She seems to visualise it by looking up to the left first and then depicting various positions of the visualised room. Now and again she looks at Brooks and stays in contact with him.

Brooks: Okay, so, that sounds to me (turning to the audience) like ... a fairly ... nasty kind of thing to have, you know. Not something you want to have, you know, for long. You want to *get rid of that one.*

> Brooks gently helps her to dissociate from the unpleasant memory and look at it. He does so by acknowledging the severity of the problem. While doing this, he turns to the audience, overtly to explain what is happening and covertly to invite her to look at the audience as well. She does so and smiles, indicating she steps out of the memory. Meanwhile, Brooks creates a link between the severity of the problem (nasty thing) and the solution (get rid of that one). Brooks also uses the technique of talking to the audience to make his suggestion indirect. To the audience, he says: "you (people in general) want to get rid of this". To her, he

indirectly says: "you (the client) want to get rid of this". He says all this in a matter-of-fact tone of voice, matching her voice tone and implying that getting rid of the problem is obvious and easy.

Embedded suggestions:

- You want to[MO] *get rid of that one.*

Embedded statements:

- Okay[DM] so[DM] that sounds to me like a fairly nasty kind of thing to have you know[DM].
- Not something you want to have, you know[DM], for long.

Vague language:

- Vague verb: get rid of
- Vague adjective: nasty
- Unspecified person: you
- Unspecified time: for long
- Unspecified object/event: nasty kind of thing, something, that one

Presuppositions:

- Qualifying adverb:
  a fairly nasty kind of thing ⊇ a nasty kind of thing

- Demonstrative determiner:
  that one ⊇ there is a specific one

Various techniques:

- Talking to others: So, that sounds to me like…
- Goal setting: You want to get rid of that one.

Brooks: Okay, and how long ago was that, a couple of weeks?

With this question, Brooks leads her attention back to the memory, but not to the content of it. Thinking and talking about the time it happened, actually helps her to dissociate further from the experience. The question is also a way of distracting her conscious from the suggestions he just gave before.

Client: That was about three weeks ago now.

Brooks: (softly) Yes.

Client: Two and a half, three weeks.

Before the client can continue, Brooks lifts his finger and turns to the audience. He moves her mind around, switching between gathering factual information, creating metaphors, joking and explaining. As such, he further depotentiates her conscious ideas and beliefs and increases the space for her unconscious mind to express itself.

Vague language:

- Unspecified time: a couple of weeks

Brooks: Now, a story (turning to the audience) <name client> just told me, actually when we were in there, was that somebody said that they were trying to find a spider for her. And then somebody else walked in, you know, a few moments later and said, "I've got ... one" meaning actually she had a four-leaf clover. And <name client> actually thought she meant spider and she... How did you feel at that moment?

Brooks here refers to an incident that happened before the session. Sharing it with the audience is an indirect way of pointing it out to her. Again, he distracts her conscious mind from the suggestions he gave her before. Moreover, he is reframing her problem. A four-leaf clover is a universal symbol of luck. Drawing her attention to this incident is a way of saying "when you think something terrible is happening, something wonderful might happen". Then he focuses her attention on her feelings at that moment. In order to determine his course of action, he needs to get an impression of her associated experience of fear: the raw material of the therapy.

Vague language:

- Nominalisation: story
- Unspecified person: somebody, they, somebody else, she

- Unspecified time: a few moments later, at that moment
- Unspecified object/event: one
- Incomplete sentence: and she...

Presuppositions:

- Question:
  how did you feel? ⊇ you had feelings

- Qualifying adverb:
  meaning actually she had a... ⊇ meaning she had a...
  actually thought... ⊇ thought...

Various techniques:

- Metaphor: finding a four-leaved clover when expecting a spider stands for something good happening when you expect something bad
- Analogue marking: pausing before the word 'one' to emphasise it.
- Talking to others: talking to the audience

Client: I lost a heartbeat, put it that way (pointing at her chest), I panicked, I just run but luckily it wasn't.

> She answers the question "How did you feel?" in a more or less dissociated way. She reports her response and the intensity of it and kind of laughs in an incongruent way.

Brooks: So you know fully well AND you, you have a definite strong feeling (pointing at his chest, she nods) whenever...

Client: Oh yeah.

Brooks: ... whenever you fear that a spider or you think there might be one there.

> Brooks now leads her from a specific account of a spider situation to her general emotional response to spiders: the focus of the therapy. Rapport is reinforced by complimenting her (you know fully well..), acknowledging the intensity of her experience (strong feeling) and

matching her body language (hand to the heart). She follows his lead, verbally ("Yeah") and nonverbally (nodding).

Adjunctive and dependent suggestions:

- You know fully well - AND you have a definite strong feeling - WHENEVER you fear that a spider…

Vague language:

- Vague verb: fear
- Vague adjective: strong
- Unspecified object/event: one, a spider
- Mind reading: you know...; you have a definite strong feeling

Presuppositions:

- Qualifying adjective:
  you have a <u>definite</u> <u>strong</u> feeling ⊇ you have a <u>strong</u> feeling ⊇ you have a feeling

- Qualifying adverb:
  you know <u>fully</u> <u>well</u> ⊇ you know <u>well</u> ⊇ you know

Various techniques:

- Complimenting: "You know fully well…"

Client: Yeah.

Brooks: Okay. Can I ask you just to do something? Can I just ask you to close your eyes in a minute?

> Brooks prepares her now for an associated experience of her fear. He repeatedly uses the word 'just', suggesting the task he is giving her is simple. He is asking her conscious mind for her cooperation (Can I ask you just to…?) while at the same time giving her unconscious mind suggestions, first a vague one (do something) then a specific one (close your eyes). The allowed delay (in a minute) gives her some freedom of choice, which makes it even easier to follow the suggestions (immediately).

Brooks: and WHEN you close your eyes (moving his hand downward before his own eyes), I would like you, just, to *imagine a spider*, AND *see how you feel*, WHEN you do that. (she closes her eyes for a few seconds).

> Brooks observes her beginning response of eye closure and continues with a presupposition (you will close your eyes) and embedded suggestion (imagine a spider). The suggestion "see how you feel" matches her familiar see-feel response: seeing a spider and then feeling fear. Brooks is now testing to what extent she can associate with her feelings just by imagining a spider. Her response will determine his course of action[47]. Deliberately provoking her fear in the therapy context also creates a subtle link between experiencing the problem and solving it.
>
> Embedded suggestions:
>
> - <u>I would like you to</u>[ER] <u>just</u>[DA] *imagine a spider.*
>
> Dependent/adjunctive suggestions:
>
> - WHEN you close your eyes - I would like you, just, to *imagine a spider* - AND *see how you feel* - WHEN you do that.
>
> Vague language:
>
> - Vague verb: imagine
> - Unspecified time: in a minute
> - Unspecified object/event: something, a spider
>
> Presuppositions:
>
> - Subordinate clause of time:
>   <u>when</u> you close your eyes $\supseteq$ you will close your eyes

Brooks: Open your eyes AND see if ***you can feel comfortable***.

> After a moment of association, Brooks leads her away from her feelings by letting her open her eyes. He also seeds a new see-feel response: "see

[47] Some people with a Spider phobia only feel fear when they see an actual spider or hallucinate one in deep trance.

- feel comfortable" that piggybacks on a simple behaviour (open your eyes).

Adjunctive suggestion:

- Open your eyes - AND see if *you can feel comfortable*

Vague language:

- Unspecified adjective: comfortable
- Permissive: you can

Client: It's, uh (pointing at chest), I can't, I can get the feeling (pointing at face), as soon as I close my eyes, I can get the feeling, I mean, I can have my eyes open and get the feeling. And I feel just so shaky and my stomach turns (pointing at stomach). As if I'm going to be sick, you know. (Brooks subtly nods his head and softly says 'hmm' while she talks).

Brooks now simply listens and acknowledges her experience. Obviously, the client can easily associate with her fear and describe it in detail. This is a good thing because the intensity of the fear she feels when thinking about a spider is a good measure of her progress during the session. At the end, the absence of fear is proof of the successful cure of her phobia.

Brooks: Okay, so if we saw a scale of 1 to 10, of how bad it is (representing a scale with his hands).

Brooks now uses scaling, asking her to indicate how bad the feeling is, between 1 and 10. By scaling she must 'think about' her feelings (dissociation) rather than actually 'feeling them'. It also makes the feelings more tangible and easier to work with. It's no longer an all or nothing situation, she is now associating her current perception of the feeling with a specific number that can change and be checked again at the end of the session to ratify the success of the therapy.

Client: (nodding) it's a 10, it's 11 (laughing uncomfortably).

Brooks: 11, okay. (Turning towards the audience) Now, it's important when you do any work like this, to get some idea, of the severity of the problem. So, I mean, having 11, gives you an illustration of how she feels about it. But we use this scale then as a reference later, to find out ... the changes that have happened for her. We are going to ***bring that right down*** (moving his right hand downwards), SO ***she feels perfectly fine***.

The overt intention here is to explain the process to the audience. The covert intention is to pace her current state (severe problem) and to orient her towards a desired state (bring that right down, feels perfectly fine). Brooks uses a pause before the interspersed suggestion "the changes that have happened" to mark it out to her unconscious mind. The last sentence:

We are going to *bring that right down* so *she feels perfectly fine.*

Seems just a rational explanation to the audience, but in fact is a complex message to the client. It involves:

- A direct and overt statement (explanation) for the audience.
- An explicit statement of confidence to the client.
- A mixture of future tense (we are going to…) and present tense (so she feels …) which is confusing for her conscious mind
- A way of seeding the idea of bringing fear down and of feeling fine to her unconscious.
- A downward movement of his hand as a nonverbal suggestion to reduce her fear.

As is often the case in Ericksonian hypnotherapy, the lines between statement and suggestion and between present and future are blurred. It's important to note that Brooks never implies any possibility of failure. Every part of his communication and interaction, however direct or indirect, is orientated towards success. There is no doubt in his mind that the client will succeed, and he communicates this with everything he says and does so that the client too believes that she will succeed.

Cause-effect link:

- We are going to *bring that right down* - SO *she feels perfectly fine.*

Embedded statements:

- <u>It's important</u>[QA] to get some idea of the severity of the problem.

- But[DM] we use this scale to find out the changes that have happened.

Vague language:

- Nominalisation: scale, work, severity, problem, illustration, reference, changes
- Vague verb: find out, happened, bring down
- Vague adjective: fine
- Loaded word: perfectly
- Unspecified person: we, you
- Unspecified time: later
- Unspecified object/event: it, this, some idea, that
- No personal pronoun (gerund): having 11
- No personal pronoun (infinitive): It's important…to get some idea

Presuppositions:

- Relative clause:
  changes that have happened ⊇ changes have happened

- Qualifying adverb:
  bring that right down ⊇ bring that down
  she feels perfectly fine ⊇ she feels fine

Various techniques:

- Talking to others: talking to the audience
- Scaling: "if we saw a scale of 1 to 10 of how bad it is"

Brooks: Okay (sighing) ... okay (turning back to the client sighing, rubbing his hands), um, now your mum said you should come along here. How did your mum hear about me or...

Here Brooks sighs a couple of times, perhaps to collect his own thoughts, perhaps to create expectancy. He decides to ask her another irrelevant question, distracting the conscious mind from suggestions he made. All the same, a question for irrelevant information can yield valuable information. Something that can be utilised later for trance induction or therapeutic change.

Client: I, umm, rang my mum up the day that I saw the spider in the cupboard, and uhm she said you got to do something about this, this is getting ridiculous, and she looked up the Yellow Pages for me and found your number in the Yellow Pages, and so I rang you up.

Brooks: So where do you live?

Client: Southend.

Brooks: You live in Southend, so you probably rang Mary, yes, and Mary referred you on to us. Well, thank you for coming all the way up here.

> The question about her background does the job of distraction but reveals no relevant information for therapy. So Brooks finishes this section by summarising her words and thanking her for coming. The words 'all the way up here' imply 'you made an effort, you must be motivated'. Thanking her reframes the situation from 'her having a problem and needing help' to 'her doing other people a favour'. This is confusing and it further depotentiates her conscious mind. It is also an indirect suggestion to switch roles. Rather than her thanking Brooks for his help, he thanks her for her presence. It is a subtle and indirect way of increasing her role in the therapy process.

Client: That's okay (smiling).

> She accepts the gratitude, thereby accepting the implications of it.

Brooks: It is. Okay, now can I ask you ... I mean, I know this is, it seems to be a problem to you, having this, BUT do you really want to ***get rid of it altogether***? (asked with a doubting tonality).

> Let's look at the sentence 'I know *this is, it seems to be* a problem to you'. Brooks seems to be correcting himself here from 'this is' to 'it seems to be' as if he has made a mistake, but he is reframing the problem from being a problem 'this is', to being a perception of a problem 'seems to be'. So, it is a deliberate mistake and a form of pacing and leading. The phrase 'this is a problem' paces her current belief, whereas 'this seems to

be' implies that this is not necessarily true, and also implies that it is not a problem to him, as he knows he can help her resolve it. Often when Brooks appears to make a mistake, either in grammar or content, it is a deliberate ploy. While the client's conscious mind is confused or busy correcting the error, the unconscious will pick up the underlying message.

Asking her if she really wants to get rid of the problem altogether, has several purposes. Firstly, it is confusing because she probably assumes this to be obvious, so it further depotentiates her conscious mind and creates a state of receptivity for what is to follow. Secondly, the word 'really' implies that part of her might want to hold on to the problem. The question challenges her to make a decision and stimulates her motivation to change. Thirdly, the word 'altogether' implies that the problem consists of several parts and that some parts of it might be positive. It gets her to review whether there may be any secondary gains or benefits from having the problem. Lastly, it reinforces the implied certainty of success because the therapist is giving her a choice of how much of the problem to remove rather than speculating on whether it is possible. This is a form of a double bind. Once she chooses to have the problem removed 'altogether' a contract then exists between client and therapist. To what extent all these purposes of the suggestion are realised depends on the client. From her observable response, the second purpose (decision and motivation) is definitely reached.

Embedded suggestions:

- Okay[DM], now[DM] can I[MO] ask you…

Adjunctive suggestion:

- It seems to be a problem to you, having this - BUT do you really want to *get rid of it altogether*?

Vague language:

- Nominalisation: problem
- Vague verb: get rid of
- Unspecified object/event: this, it

- Mind reading: it seems to be a problem for you

Implications:

- It seems to be a problem for you[48] ⊃ it is not really a problem
- Do you want to get rid of it altogether ⊃ you might want to keep a part of it

Various techniques:

- Reframing: 'it is' to 'it seems to be'
- Keeping part of the problem: "do you really want to get rid of it?"

Client: Altogether, totally. I just, I want to be able to relax in my own home, knowing that relax, even to go in the cupboard, and get the hoover out, I want to be able to do it, so I don't have to open the cupboard and look first, before I slowly get the hoover out. And then get the hoover out and look all around the hoover first. That's my, that's the start of my hoovering job. (Brooks nods and hmms while she talks)

Brooks: Yes

Brooks here simply acknowledges her story.

Client: pulling out the sofa quick slowly, just to make sure there's nothing there before I hoover up. And things like that. (Brooks: yeah)

The client consciously confirms that she wants to get rid of the problem. She also specifies her goal: to relax in her own home. Brooks picks up this keyword 'relax', and he will feed it back to her in the form of various direct and indirect suggestions.

Brooks: Yeah, it must be difficult.

Brooks paces her helplessness. By saying, "It must be difficult", he is not reinforcing her negative belief; he is simply empathising with her experience, reinforcing the yes-set and enhancing rapport.

---

[48] The more the word 'seems' is emphasised, the stronger the implication.

Client: Very, it got to a stage, umm, after… the one a couple of weeks ago that I was even looking under the bed before I got into bed. And I was pulling the bed out from the wall so that if they came out on the wall, they wouldn't get onto the bed somehow.

> The client stays in the problem state and continues the problem story. Brooks realises that more stories about her problem will not provide any more useful information and will only confirm its severity. He allows her to talk and stays in rapport by nodding and saying 'yes' but does so in a monotonous voice, so as not to encourage her to go on talking.

Brooks: Okay. Before we go any further, I want ... I want you to meet somebody, okay?

> At this point, he interrupts her story by saying "Okay" (firmly and quickly). The phrase 'before we go any further' has several implications. The obvious implication is 'we will be going further'. Also, the word 'further' ratifies the stories she has just told and connects them to the next step. Finally, the words 'we go' suggest a shift from 'her talking' to 'us going'.

Client: (looking away to the left) Yeah (softly)

Brooks: Okay?!

> Brooks notices her hesitant response to his suggestion to meet someone. He says "Okay" with a voice tone that occupies the middle ground between asking her if it is okay and telling her it is okay. He uses a single word pronounced in an ambiguous way to pace and lead her experience.
>
> Vague language:
>
> - Vague verb: meet
> - Unspecified person: we, somebody
> - Vague adverb: further
> - Mind reading: it must be difficult
>
> Presuppositions:
>
> - Subordinate clause of time:
>   <u>before</u> we go any further $\supseteq$ we'll go further

- Qualifying adverb:
  we go <u>any</u> further $\supseteq$ we go further

Brooks: Something occurred to me because she is here, uhh, that she might be able to just shed some light on ... on this, and *having the change*. Rita, would you mind sharing something? I mean, would you mind just doing that? Is it possible, you can do it from back there (pointing to her position), or up here (pointing to the stage), I don't mind (laughing). (To the client) Rita came just..., Rita was sitting in this chair (pointing to the client's chair), she is here now (pointing at Rita in the audience).

(Rita talks about her fear of spiders and how Brooks helped her to get over it. The client looks at her attentively and says "yeah" and nods several times during her story.)

> A previous client who has overcome a similar problem proves two things: the problem is solvable, and Brooks knows how to deal with it. Brooks often talks about successful therapies with previous clients, using them as an analogy for the current client. If, however, the previous client is present to tell the story, as in this case, that is even better. Saying that Rita was sitting in the same chair is another way of suggesting the similarity between the two cases. It is also a way of suggesting that sitting in that chair helps to solve the problem.

Client: (looks at Brooks again) Okay.

Brooks: Just, AS she is here, it might be interesting for you to *hear that*.

Client: Yeah.

Brooks: You know, AS A DEMONSTRATION of what *you can achieve*. (turns to the previous client) And that was what, two years ago? Something like that? Something like that. I can't remember. (Rita shares some more details about her problem)

> Now let's look at the suggestion 'what you can achieve'. Brooks doesn't say 'you can achieve the same results as Rita'. That would be direct and specific. Instead, the suggestion is vague (what you can achieve), embedded (you know...) and indirectly linked to Rita's story (as a demonstration of). His voice tone is very casual as if his remark is not

relevant. Indirect and casual remarks are easily ignored by the conscious mind, but they are picked up by the unconscious. Brooks immediately shifts to the other person and again talks about something irrelevant (when was that?). This is another way of distracting the client's conscious mind from the suggestion he has just given her.

Embedded suggestions:

- She might[MO] be able to[MO] just[DA] *shed some light.*
- It might be interesting[QA] for you to *hear that.*

Dependent suggestions:

- AS she is here - it might be interesting for you to *hear that.*

Adjunctive suggestions:

- She might be able to just shed some light on this - AND *having the change.*

Explanatory link:

- It might be interesting for you to *hear that*, you know - AS A DEMONSTRATION of what *you can achieve.*

Vague language:

- Nominalisation: demonstration
- Vague verb: occurred, achieve
- Unspecified object/event: this, something, it

Various techniques:

- Analogy: success story by a previous client

Client: Just like me.

The client recognises something in Rita's story, which makes the analogy effective.

Brooks: Hmm. So, see, what you have is fairly common, actually (Client: Yeah) BUT also (gesturing with right hand) ... change is fairly common as well (gesturing towards the previous client). It's possible to (gesturing again) ***get over it fairly easily***. That's fairly common as well.

Here, Brooks normalises her problem by defining it as fairly common. Why does he say 'fairly' common? Well, because 'fairly common' is probably easier for her conscious mind to accept than 'common'. At the same time, 'fairly common' implies 'common' and her unconscious mind will pick up that implication. So the suggestion is acceptable for the conscious and powerful for the unconscious: another example of multilevel communication. Brooks has now created a sequence of linked ideas:

Rita having the same problem → the problem is common → change is common → 'getting over it' is common/easy.

Of course, these ideas are not logically linked, and they did not exist beforehand; they are created with language.

Embedded suggestions:

- <u>It's possible</u>[MO] to *get over it fairly easily.*

Adjunctive suggestion:

- What you have is fairly common, actually - BUT also change is fairly common.

Direct statement:

- That's fairly common as well.

Vague language:

- Nominalisation: change
- Vague verb: get (over it)
- Vague adverb: fairly, easily
- Vague adjective: common
- Unspecified object/event: what you have, that
- Comparative deletion: common (no reference)
- No personal pronoun (infinitive): it's possible to get over it

Presuppositions:

- Qualifying adverb:
  get over it <u>fairly</u> <u>easily</u> ⊇ get over it <u>easily</u> ⊇ get over it

<u>fairly</u> common ⊇ common

Various techniques:

- Analogue marking: emphasising the word 'change', pausing before it, gesturing while saying it.

Client: Could you teach it again? Could you be taught it again? That's what...that's what I'm scared off.

The client here brings up what Brooks calls a roadblock: a limiting belief that stands in the way of reaching her goal. Her belief expresses her external locus of control: "something or someone might teach me to be scared again". You can notice the two different voices she uses: a high-pitched, childlike voice and a lower-pitched, adult voice. Brooks will later use a high-pitched voice when he engages the client in a play in which she becomes friends with a spider and has fun playing with it (as a child would do).

Brooks: (shaking his head) Once you, once you've learned to get over it, you won't unlearn it, you can't unlearn that.

Client: Yeah.

Brooks: You won't ... you won't be able to ... You'll always ... ONCE you're ... ONCE ***you're confident***, ONCE ***you are confident with spiders, you will never ever go back*** to how it used to be (gesturing behind the client), ***you will always be very, very confident***.

Client: (nodding) Okay.

Brooks: You can't undo that, ONCE it's happened (turning his head to the audience).

Here, Brooks answers her questions with multilevel communication. To her conscious mind, he answers her question and tells her that she cannot and will not unlearn what she will learn here, almost as if he is telling her a scientific fact. To her unconscious mind, he gives a series of embedded suggestions. Here we have a nice example of how the embedding structure of a suggestion in itself contains another suggestion and an implication. For example:

Once *you are confident*, *you will never ever go back.*

Embedded suggestion: *you will never ever go back*

Embedding structure: once *you are confident*

containing the implication: *you will be confident*

and the embedded suggestion: *you are confident*

Note that the lines between the present (you are confident) and the future (you will be confident) are blurred here. The conscious mind will not recognise this, and the unconscious mind can simply follow the suggestion *to be confident* (at any time). Brooks' voice tone shifts in the course of this piece from casual and informative to powerful and suggestive. Before, he has already defined the process of 'getting over her fear' as easy. Now he links this process to two desired states: the inability to get the fear back and permanent future confidence. Brooks uses suggestions to avoid an undesired state:

- you won't/can't unlearn it
- you won't be able to...
- you will never ever go back to how it used to be
- you can't undo that

and suggestions to achieve a desired state:

- once you're confident with spiders
- you will always be very, very confident

covering both her thinking styles: 'away from' and 'towards'.

Brooks' suggestions in this part are very direct. This is possible because the client is responsive, rapport is intense and she relies on his judgment (thinking style: external reference). Not only does he suggest confidence to the client, but he also demonstrates it as well. He speaks, moves, and acts confidently when he answers her questions. His verbal and nonverbal communication is congruent.

Dependent suggestions:

- ONCE you've learned to get over it - you won't unlearn it, you can't unlearn that, you won't be able to.
- ONCE *you are confident with spiders - you will never ever go back* to how it used to be, *you will always be very, very confident, you will never ever go back.*
- You can't undo that - ONCE it's happened.

Vague language:

- Nominalisation: confidence
- Vague verb: learn, unlearn, go back, undo
- Vague adjective: confident
- Unspecified object/event: it, that
- Universal quantifier: always, never ever

Presuppositions:

- Subordinate clause of time:
  <u>once</u> you have learned ⊇ you can/will learn
  <u>once</u> you are confident ⊇ you can/will be confident
  <u>once</u> it's happened ⊇ it can/will happen

- Qualifying adverb:
  you will always be <u>very, very</u> confident ⊇ you will always be confident

Implications:

- how it <u>used to be</u> ⊃ it is not anymore
- you will never ever <u>go</u> back ⊃ getting the problem back would be an active step, something you have control over[49]

[49] As opposed to 'falling back' which would imply having no control.

Various techniques:

- Analogue marking: gesturing behind the client to put the location of the problem in the past

The previous client shares some more about her story. The client listens to her story and laughs. The story then triggers a memory of her own, which she shares.

Client: I went into my friend's house the other day, well, about a month ago now. And she had a plastic one. Her daughter had put a plastic one in the toilet roll holder, in the actual toilet roll, and as I had gone to fetch the toilet roll, I noticed it haven't I, and I literally rushed out, my knickers down (laughing heartily) and I've legged it out of the house quick.

Brooks: (laughing) I can *see it quite clearly*.

Brooks is laughing with her, and with this remark, he enhances the humour of her story. He also tells her how to experience it: in the visual modality (see it).

Client: It sounds silly but it's true, I'll tell you. I can laugh about it now, but at the time...ha-ha.

Brooks: Yeah, you must have been very frightened.

Here, Brooks' comment ratifies the seriousness of her story and also helps her focus on the emotional aspect of it (which is her actual problem).

Client: Yeah, I killed her daughter, put it that way.

She now finishes her story and looks at him expectantly.

Brooks: Okay, what I'd like you to do... could I just (he reaches out to her right arm and she immediately offers it) hold your arm a minute? I'm going to lift your arm up, AND I'd like you to ... these rings (lifting her hand and pointing to the rings on her fingers), do they mean anything special to you, these rings here?

This is a pivotal point in the session, where Brooks actively shifts from information gathering and rapport building to induction and therapy. The word 'okay' and the pronunciation of it ratify and round off the first part of the session. His body language, a deep breath and an upward gesture signal something new coming up. He asks her if he can hold her arm and then takes it before she can answer. She responds involuntarily, even before he has finished the question. The question seems to give her a choice, but before she can really think about it, she is already experiencing it physically. The conscious mind is distracted by the question, the unconscious can experience the feeling. Brooks chooses her rings as a fixation spot for trance induction. Before he does this, he checks for possible associations she might have with them. The word 'special' is vague, and it can have a positive or negative meaning for her. Her response will determine whether or not to use the rings. In this section, Brooks uses several half sentences. He allows himself to cut off or change his statements or suggestions at any moment, often in response to the nonverbal cues from the client[50].

Embedded suggestions:

- I can[MO] *see it quite clearly.*

Adjunctive suggestions:

- I'm gonna lift your arm up - AND I'd like you to…

Vague language:

- Vague adjective: special
- Unspecified time: a minute
- Incomplete sentence: I would like you to...

Presuppositions:

- Qualifying adverb:
  see it quite clearly ⊇ see it clearly ⊇ see it
- Pseudo-cleft sentence:
  what I would like you to do... ⊇ I would like you to do something

Client: One is from my mother, and one's from my nan.

---

[50] Sometimes incomplete or dangling sentences are deliberately used to created open-ended suggestions.

Her response seems to be neutral or positive so Brooks knows he can use the rings for eye fixation. The fact that she wears rings from her mother and her grandmother confirms her family-oriented lifestyle.

Brooks: Okay, so they are quite special, in fact, aren't they? Have a look at those ... rings there (gently pushing her wrist in various directions). *Be aware of your arm in the air* like that AND look at the rings. I want you to ... can you *see the light* reflected off the stones in there at all? See the reflection, yeah.

Brooks now induces trance with a combination of eye fixation and arm catalepsy. The eye fixation occurs by having her stare at the light reflecting off the stones of her rings. The ambiguous phrase 'see the light' is a specific behavioural instruction and also a vague suggestion for her unconscious mind. While her conscious mind focuses on the stones, Brooks gently pushes her arm in various directions, thereby locking it in space.

Questions with an embedded suggestion:

- Can you *see the light* reflected off the stones?

Adjunctive suggestions:

- *Be aware of your arm in the air* like that - AND look at the rings.

Embedded statements:

- Okay[DM] so[DM] they are quite special in fact[SA] aren't they[TA]?

Vague language:

- Vague adjective: special
- Unspecified place: in the air
- Unspecified process: like that
- Incomplete sentence: I want you to...

Presuppositions:

- Qualifying adverb:
  they are quite special ⊇ they are special

- Demonstrative determiner:
  those rings ⊇ there are specific rings

Implications:

- your arm in the air <u>like that</u> ⊃ your arm is in the air in a special way

Various techniques:

- Metaphor: 'see the light from the rings' stands for 'see the light in your life'
- Induction: eye fixation and arm catalepsy
- Symbolism: rings and stones as symbols for possible resources

Client: Yeah.

Brooks: Keep your eyes on that for a moment. What I want you to ... *experience*, AS you keep your eyes on that ... ring there. At the same time, you keep your eyes on that ring, I'd like you to *think of ... how you feeeel, if you were somewhere very comfortable and special.* Like on a holiday or *somewhere you know which is a very, very nice place to be.* Where would you be? Can you *think of somewhere*?

> Here, Brooks induces a state of comfort by having her think of a familiar, comfortable place. It is also a shift from an external visual experience (the rings) to an internal visualisation (think of somewhere) and sensation (how you feel). Thinking of a nice place is made dependent (AS) on looking at the ring. The trance induction process now includes three techniques: eye fixation, arm catalepsy and visualisation.
>
> Embedded suggestions:
>
> - What <u>I want you to</u>^{ER} *experience...*
> - <u>I'd like you to</u>^{ER} *think of how you feel if you were somewhere very comfortable and special.*
> - <u>Somewhere you know</u>^{PA} which is *a very, very nice place to be.*
>
> Dependent suggestions:
>
> - What I want you to *experience* - AS you keep your eyes on that ring.
>
> Questions with an embedded suggestion:
>
> - Can you *think of somewhere*?

Vague language:

- Nominalisations: holiday
- Vague verb: experience
- Vague adjective: comfortable, special
- Unspecified time: for a moment
- Unspecified place: somewhere, on holiday, a very nice place
- Unspecified object/event: that

Presuppositions:

- Question:
  <u>where</u> would you be? ⊇ you would be somewhere

- Noun clause:
  think of <u>how you feel</u> ⊇ you feel a certain way

- Subordinate clause of time:
  <u>as</u> you keep your eyes on that ring ⊇ you will keep your eyes on that ring

- Change-of-time verb:
  <u>keep</u> your eyes on that ⊇ you already have your eyes on that

- Qualifying adverb:
  somewhere <u>very</u> comfortable ⊇ somewhere comfortable

  a <u>very</u> nice place ⊇ a nice place

- Pseudo-cleft sentence:
  <u>what</u> I want you to experience…⊇ I want you to experience something

Various techniques:

- Induction: visualisation

Client: Hmm ... on the beach.

Brooks: On the beach. *Put yourself on the beach* now, in your mind, AND keep looking at that ring AS *you are on the beach*. So *you are in two places at once, you're on the beach* (pointing beside her), AND also you're looking at that ring (pointing at her right hand).

> Brooks here starts working towards dissociation by saying "put yourself on the beach" instead of "go to the beach". He also creates a double experience of external and internal visualisation using dependent (AS) and adjunctive (AND) suggestions. The ability to be in two places at once is a trance phenomenon. This ability is implied by the instruction to do it. Telling someone to do something implies that person's ability to do so.

Brooks: Now I'd like you to also *notice*, AS you look at that ring… *notice how your arm feels. It starts to get a little bit heavier, starts being heavier*, okay. *Be aware of your breathing in the same time.*

> Brooks now draws her attention to her kinaesthetic experience, the feelings in her arm and her breathing. He suggests heaviness developing in her arm. His voice changes to a trance-like tonality; it becomes deeper, slower and his pronunciation becomes less clear. Notice the gradual nature of the suggestion:
>
> *starts to get a little bit heavier - starts being heavier*
>
> The feeling of heaviness piggybacks on the simple behaviour of looking at the ring, and it is linked to the awareness of her breathing. What's more, heaviness will occur naturally through gravity and fatigue in the course of time. All of this makes it easy - almost inevitable - for her to follow the suggestion and develop heaviness in her arm.
>
> Embedded suggestions:
>
> - So[DM] *you are in two places at once.*
> - Now I'd like you to[ER] also *notice…how your arm feels.*
>
> Direct suggestions:
>
> - *It starts to get a little bit heavier, starts being heavier.*
> - *Be aware of your breathing in the same time.*

Dependent/adjunctive suggestions:

- *Put yourself on the beach* now, in your mind - AND keep looking at that ring - AS *you are on the beach.*

Adjunctive suggestions:

- *You're on the beach* - AND also you're looking at that ring.

Dependent suggestions:

- Also *notice* - AS you look at that ring - *notice how your arm feels.*

Vague language:

- Nominalisation: mind, breathing
- Unspecified place: the beach, two places
- Comparative deletion: heavier

Presuppositions:

- Subordinate clause of time:
  as you are on the beach ⊇ you are on the beach
  as you look at that ring ⊇ you look at that ring

- Noun clause:
  notice how your arm feels ⊇ your arm feels in a certain way

- Change-of-time verb:
  keep looking at that ring ⊇ you are already looking at that ring
  starts being heavier ⊇ will continue being heavier

- Repetitive cue word:
  also you're looking at that ring ⊇ you are already looking at something else
  also notice... ⊇ you already notice something else

- Qualifying adverb:
  a little bit heavier ⊇ heavier

- Demonstrative determiner:
  that ring ⊇ there is a specific ring

Implications:

- you are in two places at once ⊃ you can be in two places at once.

Various techniques:

- Small steps: "starts to"; "a little bit heavier"
- Dissociation: "you're in two places at once"

Brooks: Because, AS *you become aware of your breathing*, ... now, I'd like you to notice also, that you can *let your mind wander around the beach*. Maybe *feel the warmth*, AS *your eyelids start to get heavy*, EACH TIME *they start to get a little heavier* AND maybe *hear the sound of the sea, coming in on to the beach. That sound of the sea* WHEN *it comes in, you can hear that in your mind*. And *other sounds you might hear by the seaside*, ... maybe *children playing or something like that. It's veery relaxing, veery comfortable*. And *the warm sun* maybe, ... *warm weather*.

At this point, Brooks develops the visualisation, describing sensory elements like the feelings and sounds of being on the beach. He connects these elements to another trance phenomenon —heaviness of the eyes— utilising her changed blinking rate and increasing difficulty in keeping her eyes open. The sensation of heaviness that has already been suggested for the arm is now extended to the eyes; this is the beginning of a gradual and natural process of eye closure. It is very different from classical hypnosis, where the hypnotist simply instructs eye closure, and the client follows the instruction. Here it is a natural interplay between the client's conscious and unconscious mind; the hypnotherapist has merely created the right conditions. Sounds at the beach are defined as relaxing and comfortable, linking an imagined sensory experience to a desired state. The word 'very' is not just an indication of the amount of relaxation and comfort. It also turns the words 'relaxing' and 'comfortable' into presuppositions: 'very relaxing' presupposes 'relaxing'. Furthermore, the word 'very' makes the suggestion sound more dramatic. Brooks casually introduces the idea of children playing, utilising the client's story about her friend's child playing with the plastic spider and seeding this idea for later usage in the session.

Embedded suggestions:

- I'd like you[ER] to notice[FV] also, that you can[MO] *let your mind wander around the beach.*
- And[DM] *other sounds you might hear by the seaside.*
- And[DM] *the warm sun* maybe, *warm weather.*

Direct suggestions:

- *It's very relaxing, very comfortable.*

Dependent suggestions:

- AS *you become aware of your breathing* now - I'd like you to notice also…
- *That sound of the sea* - WHEN *it comes in - you can hear that in your mind.*

Dependent/adjunctive suggestions:

- Maybe *feel the warmth* - AS *your eyelids start to get heavy* - EACH TIME *they start to get a little heavier* - AND maybe *hear the sound of the sea.*

Vague language:

- Nominalisation: mind, warmth, sound, weather
- Vague verb: notice, wander
- Vague adjective: comfortable, heavy, relaxing, warm
- Unspecified place: around the beach, by the seaside
- Unspecified object/event: that, it, something
- Ambiguity (homophone): let your mind wander/wonder
- Permissive: you can, maybe, you might
- Open-ended: …or something like that; ...and other sounds

Presuppositions:

- Ordinal numeral:
  each time they start to… $\supseteq$ they will start to... several times

- Subordinate clause of time:

as you become aware of…⊇ you will become aware of your breathing
as your eyelids start to get heavy ⊇ your eyelids will start to get heavy
each time they start to…⊇ they will start to…

- Change-of-time verb:
  start to get heavy ⊇ will continue to get heavy

- Repetitive cue word:
  notice also ⊇ you are already noticing things
  other sounds you might hear ⊇ you are already hearing sounds

- Qualifying adverb:
  a little heavy ⊇ heavy
  very relaxing ⊇ relaxing
  very comfortable ⊇ comfortable

Various techniques:

- Small steps: "get a little heavy"
- Sensory experience: warmth of the sun; sound of the sea

Brooks: AS *your arm starts to get a little heavier*, notice *it starts to want to lower*, BUT don't *let it lower all the way down* yet. Because WHEN *it starts to lower*, I want you to *go deeply and deeply relaxed.* EACH TIME *it lowers a little at a time*, *deeper and slowly, let your whole body relax.*

Brooks notices her arm starts to slightly lower. He utilises this by mentioning it and then frustrating it (don't let it...yet). Furthermore, he makes the arm lowering dependent on relaxation. This is typical Ericksonian hypnotherapy, to piggyback a desired state (relaxation) on an inevitable process (arm lowering). The client's conscious mind tries to follow the direct instructions (keep your arm up and your eyes open) whereas her unconscious mind picks up the implications (lower your arm and close your eyes). According to Brooks, implicit messages are usually stronger than explicit ones. This means her unconscious will 'win' and take over - and she will go into trance. The lowering of her arm and the associated relaxation is not only a deepening process, it is also a metaphor for lowering her level of fear.

Embedded suggestions:

- I want you to[ER] *go deeply and deeply relaxed.*

Dependent suggestions:

- WHEN *it starts to lower* - I want you to *go deeply and deeply relaxed.*
- EACH TIME *it lowers a little at a time, deeper and slowly - let your whole body relax.*

Dependent/adjunctive suggestions:

- AS *your arm starts to get a little heavier* - notice *it starts to want to lower* - BUT don't *let it lower all the way down* yet.

Vague language:

- Vague adverb: deeply
- Vague adjective: relaxed
- Comparative deletion: heavier, deeper

Presuppositions:

- Subordinate clause of time:
  as your arm starts to get a little heavier ⊇ your arm will start to get heavy
  when it starts to lower ⊇ it will start to lower
  each time it lowers ⊇ it will lower a number of times

- Change-of-time verb:
  it starts to want to lower ⊇ it will continue to want to lower

- Change-of-time adverb:
  don't let it lower all the way down yet ⊇ you can/will let it lower all the way down later

- Qualifying adverb:
  get a little heavier ⊇ get heavier

Various techniques:

- Small steps: "starts to"; "a little heavier"; "little at a time"
- Frustrating response: "don't let it lower all the way down yet"
- Metaphor: 'automatic lowering of an arm' stands for 'automatic lowering of fear'

Brooks: This is just the tension AND *rigidity in your arm* at this moment. Then AS *your arm starts to get heavy, you go a little deeper relaxed.* As if *you are on the beach* now. Just *going deeper relaxed, deeper, deeper.* EACH TIME you breathe out, *a little deeper relaxed.* BUT DON'T ... *allow your eyes to close aaall the way* AND *go into a nice comfortable relaxed state all the way,* UNTIL *that hand ... lowers all the way down to the chair.*

Brooks notices her tension and defines it as 'this is just the tension and rigidity in your arm at this moment'. Now, this is a very loaded sentence. Firstly, it normalises her experience of having tension. Secondly, it directs and limits the tension to the arm, implying that the rest of her body can relax. Thirdly, it links tension to rigidity, simply by using the word 'and'. Since the rigidity in her arm has been induced by Brooks, he can take it away. This means he can take her tension away too because it is linked to rigidity. Finally, the phrase 'at this moment' implies that her tension/rigidity will change. Depending on which words are emphasised[51] it could imply that the tension/rigidity will decrease or increase. Brooks' pronunciation is ambiguous and both actually will happen: her arm relaxes now when it drops down to the chair, and it becomes rigid again at the end of the session. Brooks uses the current arm catalepsy to seed the idea of a stronger catalepsy later.

Many other things happen in this section. Brooks creates a series of links using dependent and adjunctive suggestions. Relaxation is made dependent on three things: 1. being on the beach; 2. her arm getting heavy; and 3. breathing out. Eye closure is made dependent on the full lowering of the hand. In turn, eye closure is linked to a nice, comfortable, relaxed state. Brooks has now put her in a situation where whatever she does is fine. If she experiences tension, holds her arm up and keeps her

[51] Try saying the sentence emphasising either the word 'just' or the phrase 'this moment'.

eyes open, that's what he instructed. If she lowers her arm, closes her eyes, and relaxes, that's what he implied. All possible responses are defined as cooperation and will eventually lead to the same result: trance.

Embedded suggestions:

- As if[LS] *you are on the beach* now[TA].
- Just[DA] *going deeper relaxed, deeper, deeper.*

Dependent suggestions:

- AS *your arm starts to get heavy - you go a little deeper relaxed.*
- EACH TIME you breathe out - *a little deeper relaxed.*

Adjunctive suggestion:

- This is just the tension - AND *rigidity in your arm* at this moment.

Dependent/adjunctive suggestions:

- BUT DON'T *allow your eyes to close all the way* - AND *go into a nice comfortable relaxed state all the way* - UNTIL *that hand lowers all the way down.*

Vague language:

- Nominalisation: tension, rigidity, state
- Vague verb: go deeper, allow
- Vague adjective: heavy, a little, deeper, relaxed, comfortable, down, all the way, nice, comfortable, relaxed
- Unspecified time: at this moment
- Unspecified object/event: this
- Comparative deletion: deeper
- No personal pronoun: (gerund) just going deeper relaxed

Presuppositions:

- Change-of-time verb:
  starts to get heavy $\supseteq$ get heavy

- Qualifying adjective:

a <u>nice</u> <u>comfortable</u> relaxed state ⊇ a <u>comfortable</u> relaxed state ⊇ a relaxed state

- Qualifying adverb:
  close your eyes <u>all the way</u> ⊇ close your eyes
  <u>a little</u> <u>deeper</u> relaxed ⊇ <u>deeper</u> relaxed ⊇ relaxed
  lowers <u>all the way</u> down ⊇ lowers down

- Demonstrative determiner:
  <u>that</u> hand ⊇ there is a specific hand

Implications:

- this is <u>just</u> the tension…⊃ the tension is not a problem
- the tension…<u>at this moment</u> ⊃ the tension will change

Various techniques:

- Frustrating response: "<u>don't</u> allow your eyes to close and... <u>until</u>..."

Brooks: Just *let it go slowly*, that's it, you are doing very well. Just *deeper relaxed, deeper relaxed, and deeper relaxed.* That's it, doing very well. Just *deeper, ... deeper.* And part of you almost wants it to *lower ... faster than that*, BUT just *keep it ... lowering sloowly.* Anyway, this part of you probably wants to *close your eyes.* Just keep them open a little longer, that's it. EACH TIME *you blink*, maybe *get a bit heavier.* And it's that feeling like *you want to close them*, BUT ... I'm asking you to keep them open just a bit longer UNTIL *they just can't wait* anymore AND *they have to close*, AS *you go deeper* and *deeper relaxed, deeper.*

> Her arm has gone down most of the way, and her eyes are almost closed now. Brooks compliments her on this and becomes a little more direct in his deepening suggestions. He is still frustrating her desired response of closing her eyes, making it all the more compelling. At the same time, he is pacing and encouraging her unconscious (part of you) to continue this behaviour. By asking for only small responses (a bit heavier, a little longer), he makes it very easy for her to follow. The suggestion "I'm asking you to keep them open…until…they have to close" links the instruction to keep her eyes open to the necessity of closing them and

going deeper. The client is in a double bind: whatever she does leads to eye closure and trance.

Embedded suggestions:

- Just[DA] *let it go slowly.*
- Just[DA] *deeper relaxed, deeper relaxed and deeper relaxed.*
- Just[DA] *deeper, deeper.*
- Just[DA] *keep it lowering slowly.*
- Anyway[DM] this part of you probably wants to[MO] *close your eyes.*
- Just[DA] keep them open a little longer.

Dependent suggestions:

- EACH TIME you blink - maybe *get a bit heavier.*

Adjunctive suggestions:

- Part of you almost wants it to *lower faster than that* - BUT just *keep it lowering slowly.*

Dependent/adjunctive suggestions:

- *You want to close them* - BUT I'm asking you to keep them open just a bit longer - UNTIL *they just can't wait anymore* - AND *they have to close* - AS *you go deeper* and *deeper relaxed.*

Vague language:

- Vague adjective: relaxed
- Vague adverb: slowly
- Unspecified object/event: it, part of you
- Comparative deletion: deeper, longer, heavier
- No personal pronoun (gerund): *doing* very well
- Permissive: probably, maybe

Presuppositions:

- Change-of-time verb:
  keep it lowering $\supseteq$ you are already lowering it

- Qualifying adverb:

let it go <u>slowly</u> ⊇ let it go
<u>a bit</u> heavier ⊇ heavier
<u>a bit</u> longer ⊇ longer

- Subordinate clause of time:
  <u>each time</u> you blink ⊇ you will blink a number of times

- Demonstrative determiner:
  <u>this</u> part of you ⊇ there is a specific part of you (your unconscious)
  <u>that</u> feeling ⊇ there is a specific feeling

Various techniques:

- Complimenting: ”you are doing very well”
- Ratifying nonverbal response: “that’s it“
- Frustrating response: ”keep them open just a little bit longer”
- Conscious-unconscious dissociation: ”*this part of you* wants to close your eyes”; ”just keep them open”
- Small steps: “a bit/little longer”; “a bit heavier”

Brooks: Doing very well, just *deeper ... and deeper ...* And you can wonder whether *you go aaaalll the way down* (she closes her eyes now), *into a nice deeeep comfortable, relaxed state*, before it touches your arm. That’s it, *all the way down.* (Her arm is probably on the armrest now) Just *allow your arm to relax* now. (she is leaning her head against the chair) You can *let your head relax*, that’s it, *all the way back*. And ***feel nice and comfortable***, thaaaat’s it. Doing very well, doing very, very well indeed. Just *relaxing* AND *hear the sound of my voice*, AND the sound of an ice-cream van in the distance.

> Brooks compliments her while giving more deepening suggestions. He uses another double bind, giving her the options of “going all the way down” before or after her arm touches. Then he utilises her spontaneous head movement by suggesting it (“you can let your head relax”). This gives her permission for her behaviour but, more importantly, it connects her behaviour to his words. Brooks often uses this technique of suggesting a response that has just occurred or that has just started. It brings the behaviour under his ‘control’. The suggestion “hear the *sound*

of my voice" implies "don't listen to the words". Her conscious mind can hear the sound, while her unconscious hears the words. Brooks utilises the external sound of an ice cream van by linking it to the sound of his voice and suggesting it to be 'in the distance'[52].

Embedded suggestions:

- Just[DA] *deeper and deeper.*
- And[DM] you can[MO] wonder[EQ] whether *you go all the way down into a nice deep comfortable relaxed state.*
- Just[DA] *allow your arm to relax* now[TA].
- You can[MO] *let your head relax*, that's it, *all the way back.*
- And[DM] *feel nice and comfortable.*

Adjunctive suggestions:

- *Just relaxing* - AND *hear the sound of my voice* - AND the sound of an ice-cream van in the distance.

Vague language:

- Nominalisation: distance
- Vague verb: go deeper, wonder, relaxing
- Vague adjective: deep, relaxed, nice, comfortable
- Vague adverb: well
- Unspecified place: in the distance
- Unspecified object/event: it
- Comparative deletion: deeper
- No personal pronoun (gerund): *doing* very well; just *relaxing*

Presuppositions:

- Subordinate clause of time:
  before it touches $\supseteq$ it will touch

- Double bind:

[52] The sound of an ice cream van might also elicit positive childhood memories.

whether you go all the way down before it touches your arm (or after) $\supseteq$ you will go all the way down

- Change-of-time adverb:
  they just can't wait anymore $\supseteq$ they have been waiting for a long time

- Qualifying adverb:
  very well $\supseteq$ well
  all the way down $\supseteq$ down

- Qualifying adjective:
  a nice deep comfortable relaxed state $\supseteq$ a relaxed state

Implications:

- hear the sound of my voice $\supset$ don't hear the words

Various techniques:

- Complimenting: "doing very well"
- Ratifying nonverbal response: "that's it"

Brooks: AS *you experience* maybe *some fluttering in your eyelids*, *some movements in your eyelids*, realise that *that fluttering and moving in your eyelids can help you ... with your problem.* You might wonder how *that can happen.* That ... *that movement and the fluttering in your eyelids* IS SO CHARACTERISTIC OF a good hypnotic subject. Someone who can *just relaaaax* AND *really benefit from this experience* AND *learn to get over the problem quickly. Learn to leave that problem in the past* (gesturing to a spot behind her), AND just to *move ahead into the future* (gesturing to a spot before her), *in a new freedom* from the old problem. How nice, to be able, to *do that.* Just *enjoy being on that beach now.*

Brooks observes the fluttering of her eyelids and her eye movement and utilises it by suggesting that this will help her benefit from the session. He also defines the fluttering as characteristic of a good hypnotic subject. So he has now created the link:

fluttering eyelids → trance → therapeutic change

Her conscious mind will accept this as information about how the process 'works'. Her unconscious mind will pick this up as a suggestion about how to 'make it work'. Brooks will come back to this link about 10 minutes later in the session. The suggestion "you might wonder how that can happen" is a nice example of multi-level communication. On one level, it is a statement to pace any conscious curiosity or doubt. On another level, it is a suggestion to unconsciously make this happen. Defining the fluttering as "characteristic of a good hypnotic subject" is an indirect compliment. Praising the client for being a good hypnotic subject is a technique Brooks often uses. It is very different from classical hypnosis where the hypnotisability of the client is considered to be a fixed, predetermined condition. Brooks compliments the client for 'being' a good hypnotic subject in order to 'make' her a better hypnotic subject. Hypnotisability is not considered to be a fixed trait of the client, but a flexible response that depends on the client, the hypnotist, and the level of rapport between them. Note that the compliment is also a change in logical levels (Dilts R. B., 1999) from positive behaviour (trance behaviour) to positive identity (a good hypnotic subject). Brooks immediately links this new identity to a series of suggested abilities:

> Someone who can *just relax, really benefit from the experience, learn to get over the problem quickly…*

This serial suggestion is then casually repeated and summarised with an indirect suggestion:

> How nice, to be able, to *do that.*

After a flood of suggestions for relaxation, deepening, learning and change, Brooks distracts her conscious mind by inviting it to 'enjoy being on the beach'.

Embedded suggestions:

- Realise[FV] that *that fluttering and moving in your eyelids can help you.*
- You might[MO] wonder[EQ] how *that can happen.*
- How nice[QA] to be able[MO] to *do that.*
- Just[DA] *enjoy being on the beach* now[TA].

Dependent suggestions:

- AS *you experience* maybe *some fluttering in your eyelids* - realise that *that fluttering and moving in your eyelids can help you.*

Adjunctive suggestions:

- Someone who can *just relax* - AND *really benefit from this experience* - AND *learn to get over the problem quickly.*
- Learn to *leave that problem in the past* - AND just to *move ahead into the future, in a new freedom.*

Explanatory link:

- *That movement and the fluttering in your eyelids* - IS SO CHARACTERISTIC OF a good hypnotic subject.

Vague language:

- Nominalisation: movement, problem, freedom
- Vague verb: experience, realise, help, wonder, relax, benefit, learn, leave, move ahead, enjoy
- Vague adjective: characteristic, new, old
- Loaded word: freedom
- Unspecified person: a good hypnotic subject, someone
- Unspecified time: in the past, the future
- Unspecified object/event: some fluttering, some movements
- No personal pronoun (infinitive): how nice *to be able* to do that
- Ambiguity (homophone): ahead (figuratively) or a head (literally)
- Mind reading: you might wonder…
- Permissive language: maybe, you might

Presuppositions:

- Embedded question:
  <u>you might wonder how</u> that can happen ⊇ that can happen

- Qualifying adjective:
  a <u>new</u> freedom ⊇ a freedom

- Qualifying adverb:
  someone who can <u>just</u> relax ⊇ someone who can relax
  <u>really</u> benefit from this experience ⊇ benefit from this experience
  <u>sooo</u> characteristic ⊇ characteristic

- Demonstrative determiner:
  <u>that</u> fluttering ⊇ there is a specific fluttering
  <u>that</u> movement ⊇ there is a specific movement

Various techniques:

- Complimenting: "...is so characteristic of *a good hypnotic subject*"
- Mentioning observable physical responses: "as you experience maybe some fluttering in your eyelids"

Brooks: And you know, you can *be aware* AS *you are on the beach, of the feelings in your arms, in your legs, in your shoulders.* ... You know, *the warm sun can shine* now AND *you can be in the sun or in the shade*, it is entirely up to you. Just *be aware which part of your body feels the warmest* at the moment, *which part of your body has the warmth.* Just *be aware of that.* Is it your arms or your legs?

> Brooks continues the deepening process, focusing her on physical feelings and connecting them with the visualised experience of being on the beach. By asking which body part is the warmest, he implies that one part is warmer than another. He puts her into a double bind, giving her the illusionary choice of where to feel the warmth: in her arms, or in her legs. His voice tone remains constant during this last sentence; if he had wanted to restrict her choices to arms and legs, his voice would have gone down at the word 'legs'. Now, his voice stays at the same pitch, which suggests the sentence is not finished and she can feel the warmth in other parts of the body.

Client: My head.

> Leaving the place of warmth open was a good choice since she feels it in her head. If she hadn't sensed that openness in his voice tone, she might have been insecure about feeling it in a place other than the suggested options.

Brooks: Your head, okay. That's usually the case, anyway.

Brooks fully accepts her choice by repeating and acknowledging her words. He also normalises her experience ("okay, that's usually the case"), just in case she still feels any insecurity about her experience. Note the short pause between the words 'case' and 'anyway'. The word 'anyway' is marked out and becomes an ambiguous word that can be heard as:

- anyway: a discourse marker embedding the phrase "that's usually the case" or
- any way: suggesting various ways (places) to experience warmth.

Embedded suggestions:

- And[DM] you know[DM] you can[MO] *be aware…of the feelings in your arms.*
- Just[DA] *be aware which part of your body feels the warmest* at the moment[TA].
- Just[DA] *be aware of that.*

Dependent suggestions:

- You can *be aware* - AS *you are on the beach* - *of the feelings in your arms.*

Adjunctive suggestions:

- *The warm sun can shine* now - AND *you can be in the sun or in the shade.*

Embedded statements:

- That's usually the case anyway[DM].

Vague language:

- Nominalisation: warmth
- Unspecified time: at the moment
- Unspecified object/event: that
- Ambiguity (Homophone): anyway/any way
- Permissive: you can
- Covering all possibilities: you can be in the shade or in the sun

Presuppositions:

- Noun clause:
  be aware <u>which part of your body feels the warmest</u> ⊇ some part of your body feels the warmest

- Qualifying adverb:
  it is <u>entirely</u> up to you ⊇ it is up to you

- Double bind:
  is it <u>your arms or your legs</u> ⊇ it is some part of your body

Implications:

- which part of your body feels the warmest <u>at the moment</u> ⊃ a different part might feel the warmest later

Various techniques:

- Normalising: "that's usually the case"

Brooks: Just *be aware of that warmth in your head.* And you know, the *warmer ... you feel*, you can just *get as warm as you want*, just, BUT no warmer than is necessary for you to *feel nice and comfortable.* Really *just sooo comfortable.* You know, *aaaall worries and tensions can just drift away from your body*, just *drift away from the body.* Just *leaving you feeling nice and comfortable and relaxed.* EACH TIME you breathe, just *going deeper relaxed*, a little at a time, *nice and comfortable, deeeeper relaxed.* Just *deeeeper relaxed.* You're doing very, very well. Just *deeper relaxed*, EACH TIME you breathe out. You know *you are going to feel more relaxed than you have for a long time. So relaxed ...* you might even *surprise yourself ... what you manage to do for yourself* here today.

Brooks now utilises the warmth in her head to enhance relaxation and deepen the trance. First, he uses a permissive suggestion: 'it *can be* as warm as you want'. This tells her she has both the *freedom* and the *power* to control the warmth in her head. Then he tells her: 'but no warmer than...'. This seems to limit her freedom, but, actually it confirms her power by implication, just as the warning 'don't run more than 10 miles', for example, implies 'you can run more than 10 miles'. A certain amount of warmth is defined as necessary for feelings of comfort and relaxation, but the exact temperature is not specified; it is left for her to decide. The connection between warmth in her head and comfort is not strictly logical but probably acceptable for her conscious mind. The message for the unconscious is simple: "be as warm as you want" and "be comfortable and relaxed". After carefully setting up these connections between warmth, breathing and relaxation, Brooks suggests she can be more relaxed than she has been in a long time. Of course, 'a long time' is a vague term. It allows her to choose how long that is and how relaxed she will be accordingly. Finally, her relaxation is defined as an example of "what you manage to do for yourself". The word *what* is unspecific. Her conscious mind will logically connect it to her *relaxation* whereas her unconscious can relate that to *anything she can manage to do for herself.* The last sentence is also another step of handing over control and responsibility to the client and a way of seeding therapeutic steps that she will take later. Earlier, Brooks created the link:

> fluttering eyelids –> trance –> therapeutic change

Now he has created another one:

> warmth in the head and breathing → comfort and relaxation → doing things for yourself

Embedded suggestions:

- Just[DA] *be aware of that warmth in your head.*
- And[DM] you know[DM] the *warmer you feel…*
- You can[MO] just[DA] *get as warm as you want.*
- Really[SA] *just so comfortable.*
- You know[DM] *all worries and tensions can just drift away from your body.*
- Just[DA] *leaving you feeling nice and comfortable and relaxed.*
- Just[DA] *deeper relaxed.*
- You know[DM] *you are going to feel more relaxed than you have for a long time.*
- You might[MO] even *surprise yourself what you manage to do for yourself* here[PA] today[TA].

Dependent suggestions:

- EACH TIME you breathe - just *going deeper relaxed* a little at a time, *nice and comfortable*, *deeeeper relaxed.*
- Just *deeper relaxed* - EACH TIME you breathe out.

Adjunctive suggestions:

- You can just *get as warm as you want* - BUT no warmer than is necessary for you to *feel nice and comfortable.*

Vague language:

- Nominalisation: warmth, worries, tension
- Vague verb: drift, leaving, surprise, manage
- Vague adjective: nice, comfortable
- Loaded word: surprise
- Unspecified time: for a long time
- Unspecified object/event: that
- Unspecified quantity: a little
- Comparative deletion: warmer, deeper
- Ambiguity of meaning, scope and punctuation: worries and tensions can just drift away...*leaving you* feeling nice and comfortable and relaxed.
- Permissive: you can, you might

Presuppositions:

- Noun clause:
  surprise yourself <u>what you manage to do</u> ⊇ you manage to do something

- Qualifying adverb:
  <u>so comfortable</u> ⊇ comfortable
  <u>even</u> surprise yourself ⊇ surprise yourself

- Superlative adjective:
  part feels the <u>warmest</u> ⊇ other parts feel less warm

- Demonstrative determiner:

that warmth ⊇ there is a specific warmth

Implications:

- what you manage to do ⊃ what you do is not easy

Various techniques:

- Complimenting: "you're doing very, very well"
- Frustrating response: "but no warmer than…"
- Small steps: "starts to"; "a little at a time"

Brooks: Now you don't ... have to know ... BUT you know, things have already started to change. And you might *wonder how that has happened.* Simply by us talking, things have started to happen. Now the part of you that's *allowing you to relaaaaaax, deeper and deeper* now ... is also the part of you that is *going to help you in the future*, ***feel perfectly okay in the future****. You don't have to think about that at all* now. Just that part of you is *going to help you in ways that might surprise you, in a way, you'll be delighted with.*

The client is following Brooks' suggestions. He points this out with a vague statement: 'things have already started to change'. Mentioning signs of trance (vaguely or specifically) is a typical way of thanking or praising the unconscious and encouraging it to continue. Brooks utilises her signs of relaxation to enhance the dissociation between her conscious mind ('you' don't have to know) and unconscious mind (but 'you' know). The unconscious mind is then defined as 'the part of you that...', enhancing further dissociation. Let's look a little closer at the statement "Now the part of you that's allowing you to relax, deeper and deeper now, is also the part of you that is going to help you in the future". For the conscious mind, this is an explanation of how the process works. For the unconscious mind, however, it is a three-step suggestion: 1) You created relaxation; 2) relax deeper, and 3) you will provide help with the problem. This is a nice piece of multilevel communication and of pacing and leading. At the end of this section, conscious/unconscious dissociation is further enhanced with the suggestion "...in ways that might surprise you". Being surprised implies that something has happened to you rather than you have done it yourself.

Embedded suggestions:

- And[DM] you might[MO] *wonder how that has happened.*
- Now[DM] the part of you, that is *allowing you to relax, deeper and deeper* now[TA] is also the part of you that is *going to help you in the future, feel perfectly okay in the future.*
- *You don't have to think about that at all* now[TA].
- Just[DA] that part of you *is going to help you in ways that might surprise you, in a way, you'll be delighted with.*

Adjunctive suggestions:

- Now you don't have to know - BUT you know things have already started to change.

Cause-effect link:

- BY us talking - things have started to happen.

Vague language:

- Nominalisation: ways
- Vague verb: change, wonder, happen, help, surprise
- Vague adjective: delighted
- Loaded word: perfectly, surprise, delighted
- Unspecified time: in the future
- Unspecified object/event: things, that
- Unspecified process: in ways
- Comparative deletion: deeper
- Mind reading: you might wonder…
- Permissive: you might

Presuppositions:

- Embedded question:
  you might wonder how that has happened $\supseteq$ that has happened
- Relative clause:
  the part of you that is allowing you to relax $\supseteq$ a part of you is allowing you to relax

the part of you <u>that</u> is going to help ⊇ a part of you is going to help you

- Change-of-time verb:
  things have already <u>started</u> to change ⊇ they will go on changing
  things have <u>started</u> to happen ⊇ they will go on happening

- Change-of-time adverb:
  things have <u>already</u> started to change ⊇ things started to change sooner than expected

- Demonstrative determiner:
  <u>that</u> part of you ⊇ there is a specific part of you

- Qualifying adverb:
  <u>simply</u> by us talking ⊇ by us talking
  feel <u>perfectly</u> okay ⊇ feel okay
  don't have to think about that <u>at all</u> ⊇ don't have to think about that
  is going to help you <u>in ways that might surprise you</u> ⊇ is going to help you

Various techniques:

- Observing/utilising minimal cues: "things have already started to change"
- Amnesia gap: "in the future ... "in the future"
- Conscious, unconscious dissociation: "*you* don't have to know, but *you* know"; "*that part of you* that's allowing you"
- Downplaying the conscious mind: "you don't have to know"; "you don't have to think about that"

Brooks: What I'd like you to do, AS *you lie on the beach*, here now, just to *find a cloud*, just to *look out in the sky*. Some cloud up there, and it is to your left or to your right? Let me know when you can *see that cloud*. Can you *see that cloud?*

Client: Hmm.

Brooks: Yeah? Okay, is it over to the left (pointing to her left) or the right (pointing to her right) at this moment?

Client: To the left.

Brooks: To the left. Look up to the left AND *see that cloud.*

Client: Hmm.

Here Brooks starts to set up the imaginary context for the process of double dissociation, in this case, V/K dissociation, the separation of her inner images from her feelings. He will combine this with the conscious-unconscious dissociation he has already created. Brooks does not use the standard NLP cinema metaphor for double dissociation here. Instead, he utilises her favourite place of relaxation—the beach—and the elements available there. He chooses clouds as a projection screen and leaves her the choice of where to see them. Obviously, the choice of any location, left or right, presupposes seeing a cloud, which is the first step in the process of double dissociation. In following the steps of this process she will later look at herself, looking at herself. Right now, she experiences herself on the beach, looking at a cloud in the sky.

Embedded suggestions:

- What I'd like you to do[ER], as *you lie on the beach* here[PA] now[TA], just[DA] to *find a cloud,* just[DA] to *look out in the sky.*
- You can[MO] *see that cloud.*

Dependent suggestions:

- What I'd like you to do - AS *you lie on the beach* here now - just to *find a cloud.*

Adjunctive suggestions:

- *Look up to the left* - AND *see that cloud.*

Questions with an embedded suggestion:

- Can you *see that cloud?*

Instructions with an embedded suggestion:

- Let me know when you can *see that cloud.*

Vague language:

- Nominalisation: moment
- Unspecified place: here, in the sky, up there
- Unspecified object/event: some cloud

Presuppositions:

- Noun clause:
  let me know <u>when you can see that cloud</u> ⊇ you will be able to see that cloud

- Demonstrative determiner:
  <u>that</u> cloud ⊇ there is a specific cloud

- Double bind:
  Is it <u>to your left or to your right</u>? ⊇ it is somewhere

Implications:

- is it over to the left or the right <u>at this moment</u> ⊃ it might be somewhere else later

Brooks: This is a very special cloud. Have you ever seen a laser show, where they *project things on the clouds*?

Client: Mmm

Brooks: Mmmm, well you know you can *project things on this cloud*, which is a lovely thing to do. Because you know ... not only can you *switch the projection on*, BUT ***you can switch it off.*** So I'd like you to *imagine you've got a kind of laser by your side.* And you can just *switch on the laser* now AND you can just *watch the show on the cloud.* Just *put those lasers on the cloud* now AND *watch that happen.* Just *see that* now for yourself. *See that ... that light show in the sky, the colours and the lines and the shapes.* Just *watch that* now AS I'm talking to you. (7 sec.) And the wonderful thing about this is that it's all yours, this special place. This cloud is all yours, AND ***you can do whatever you want*** *with it.*

Defining the cloud as a *special* cloud creates curiosity. How is it special? The word *special* also associates the imaginary cloud with the (real) ring on her finger, which was also defined as special. This creates an implication that the cloud is real and that it is hers, just like the ring. Brooks gives her a brief moment to wonder and then continues by explaining how it is special. This is a typical Brooks technique; creating curiosity or expectation and then suggesting the experience you want the client to have. Later in the session, he will have her visualise a spider, but, first he sets up a positive scene that is under her control. The cloud is now explicitly defined as being hers, as is the laser. Being in control of the laser is a metaphor for being in control of the therapeutic process and of her problem.

Embedded suggestions:

- Well[DM] you know[DM] you can[MO] *project things on this cloud* which is a lovely thing to do[QA].
- Because[DM] you know[DM] not only can you *switch the projection on.*
- So[DM] I'd like you to[ER] *imagine you've got a kind of a laser by your side.*
- Just[DA] *see that* now[TA].
- You can[MO] *do whatever you want.*

Direct suggestions:

- *See that light show in the sky, the colours and the lines and the shapes.*

Dependent suggestions:

- Just *watch that* now - AS I'm talking to you.

Adjunctive suggestions:

- Not only can you *switch the projection on* - BUT *you can switch it off.*
- You can just *switch on the laser* now - AND *watch the show on the cloud.*
- Just *put those lasers on the cloud* now - AND *watch that happen.*
- This cloud is all yours - AND *you can do whatever you want with it.*

Questions with an embedded suggestion:

- Have you ever seen a laser show, where they *project things on the clouds?*

Embedded statements:

- The wonderful thing about this is[NP] that it's all yours, this special place.

Direct statements:

- This is a very special cloud.

Vague language:

- Nominalisation: show
- Vague verb: imagine, happen
- Vague adjective: lovely, wonderful
- Unspecified place: by your side, special place
- Unspecified object/event: things, colours, lines, shapes, it
- Universal quantifier: it's *all* yours
- Ambiguities: to switch on/off
- Permissive: you can

Presuppositions:

- Qualifying adjective:
  a lovely thing to do $\supseteq$ a thing to do

  kind of a laser $\supseteq$ a laser

- Demonstrative determiner:
  this cloud $\supseteq$ there is a specific cloud
  those lasers on the cloud $\supseteq$ there are specific lasers
  that light show $\supseteq$ there is a specific light show
  this special place $\supseteq$ there is a specific special place

- Noun-preposition:
  the wonderful thing about this is that it's all yours $\supseteq$ there is something wonderful about this

Various techniques:

- Metaphor: 'switching on and off the laser' stands for 'switching on and off her fear'

Brooks: And I'd like you to … *learn something else* ... of interest. And that is that you can *float up, out of your body* ... AND *stand back, up from the beach* AND *see yourself lying down on the beach looking up at the cloud* (gesturing in the directions he mentions). Just *do that now.* Just *allow yourself to float up out of your body.* It can *be a very peaceful comfortable relaxed ... feeling.* And just *look and see yourself there ... looking up at the cloud.* Let me know when you can *see that now.* (5 sec.) *There she is there.*

Client: Mmm.

Brooks: Do you like what you see?

Client: Mmm.

Brooks: Mmmmm, just *watch her there now.*

> Now the process of dissociation is taken one step further by instructing her to float out of her body and look at herself. Double dissociation can be a difficult task, but Brooks' gentle voice tone and his use of the word 'just' several times imply that it is easy. Let's look at the sentence "Let me know when you can *see that now*". For the conscious mind, this is a simple instruction to let him know something. The unconscious mind, on the other hand, will pick up on the implication of "when you can see that" being "you can see that". It will also hear the embedded suggestion at the end of the sentence "*see that now*". With the double dissociation, another version of herself has now been created. She is looking at herself lying on the beach and looking up at the cloud. Alongside her ability to control the laser, a safe context has been set up for introducing the problem (seeing spiders) at a later point.
>
> Embedded suggestions:
>
> - And[DM] I'd like you to[ER] *learn something else.*
> - Just[DA] *do that* now[TA].
> - Just[DA] *allow yourself to float up out of your body.*
> - It can[MO] *be a very peaceful comfortable relaxed feeling.*
> - And[DM] just[DA] *look and see yourself there, looking up at the cloud.*
> - Just[DA] *watch her there* now[TA].

Direct suggestions:

- *There she is there.*

Adjunctive suggestions:

- You can *float up, out of your body* - AND *stand back, up from the beach* - AND *see yourself lying down on the beach.*

Instructions with an embedded suggestion:

- Let me know when you can *see that now.*

Vague language:

- Nominalisation: interest
- Vague verb: learn
- Vague adjective: peaceful, comfortable, relaxed
- Unspecified person: she
- Unspecified place: back, up from the beach
- Unspecified object/event: something else, that
- Permissive: you can

Presuppositions:

- Noun clause:
  do you like what you see? ⊇ you see something
  let me know when you can see that ⊇ you will be able to see that

- Qualifying adjective:
  learn something else of interest ⊇ learn something else

- Repetitive cue word:
  I'd like you to learn something else ⊇ you already learned something

Various techniques:

- Dissociation: "*seeing yourself* lying down on the beach looking up at the cloud"

Brooks: What I'd like you to do AS you *watch <name client> down on the beach*, I'd like you to *help her*. Are you willing to *help her*?

Client: Mmm.

Brooks: Okay, I'd like you to *help her ... get over some problems that she has.* And ALTHOUGH they seemed major problems in the past, they are actually quite minor BECAUSE they are very easy to get over. I'd like you to be able to *help me help her.* So together *we can both help her*, the moment *she is lying on the beach looking up at the cloud, seeing that laser show up there.* That's it, up there (saying the word 'cloud' and the phrase 'up there' in a high-pitched voice).

> The double dissociation is enhanced by calling the person on the beach by name, almost as if she is watching someone else. Now, the dissociated version of herself in the sky is suggested to help 'her on the beach'. Brooks is building on his earlier suggestion of the unconscious mind helping her. He makes it very easy for her to follow his suggestion of helping herself. First, he repeats the idea of the problem being minor and easy to solve. Then he brings himself into the equation; helping herself only means helping him to help her. Let's look at the statement "although they seemed major problems in the past, they are actually quite minor because they are very easy to get over". Brooks does not tell her directly that her problem is minor. That could make her feel embarrassed or insulted, and he could lose rapport. Instead, it helps her to accept this idea in the following three-step suggestion:
>
> Although they <u>seemed</u> major problems in the past...
>
> > This is a statement that matches her idea (major problems) but implies the opposite; that the problems only <u>seem</u> major implies that they are not major.
>
> they are <u>actually</u> <u>quite</u> minor...
>
> > Now the problems are explicitly called minor, while the words <u>actually</u> and <u>quite</u> distract conscious attention away from this word.
>
> because they are very easy to get over
>
> > This link 'explains why' her problems are minor and suggests that they are easy to get over. The explanation satisfies any conscious curiosity and also resolves possible shame about experiencing

her fear as major; she didn't know it was easy to solve! Considered logically, Brooks' explanation is questionable here, but the client's conscious mind will probably accept it as a fact. Her unconscious mind will simply pick up the implied messages: 'the problem is minor and easy to get over'.

Embedded suggestions:

- Okay[DM], I'd like you to[ER] *help her get over some problems.*
- I'd like you to[ER] be able to[MO] *help me help her.*
- So[DM] together we can[MO] *both help her,* the moment[TA] *she is lying on the beach looking up at the cloud, seeing that laser show up there.*

Dependent suggestions:

- What I'd like you to do - AS you *watch <name client> down on the beach* - I'd like you to *help her.*

Adjunctive suggestion and cause-effect link:

- ALTHOUGH they seemed major problems in the past - they are actually quite minor -BECAUSE they are very easy to get over.

Questions with an embedded suggestion:

- Are you willing to *help her?*

Vague language:

- Nominalisation: problems
- Vague verb: help, get over
- Vague adjective: major
- Unspecified time: in the past, the moment
- Unspecified place: up there

Presuppositions:

- Subordinate clause of time:
  the moment she is lying on the beach ⊇ she will be lying on the beach

- Qualifying adverb:

quite minor ⊇ minor

very easy to get over ⊇ easy to get over ⊇ to get over

- Pseudo-cleft sentence:
  what I'd like you to do ⊇ I'd like you to do something

Various techniques:

- Ratifying nonverbal response: "that's it"
- Requesting commitment: "are you willing to help her? "
- Dissociation: "you help *her*"

Brooks: Hmmm, and you know with the laser, *you can write with a laser.* Have you ever seen that done? (making writing movements in the air). People, they like, *write words.*

Client: Mmm

Brooks: Mmm, I want you to *see it write the letter S on the cloud. You watch her looking up at the cloud write the letter S.* (5 sec.) You *see that letter S appear on the cloud?*

Client: Yes

Brooks: Mmm, Mmm, that's it. What I'd like you also to do, *with your mind* you know, what you can *do with your mind,* is you can *switch that laser off.* So *stay back here* (pointing behind her) AND *look at her lying on the beach* (pointing in front of her). And you just have to, *with your mind,* you just have to *say* ... *"off".* WHEN you *say "off" that laser will go off.* Just *think it to yourself in your mind* now AND *watch the laser goes off.* (7 sec.) That's it, have you done that?

Client: Yeah.

Brooks: Now *say "on"* AND *watch it go on again.* (6 sec.) There *it goes on again* (directing his voice upwards).

> So, double dissociation has been set up, the problem has been defined as minor, and a frame of cooperation has been established. Telling the client to switch the laser off and on increases her sense of control over the process. Switching off the laser also seeds the idea of switching off her fear. Step by step, the actual problem, her phobia, is introduced now and the process of hypnotic desensitisation starts. First Brooks has her

see the word 'spider', from a doubly dissociated position by spelling the word out, beginning with the letter S. The word SPIDER is really, just a symbol representing a spider, and the letter S is just a fraction of that symbol. Controlling the laser is now a metaphor for regulating her feelings, and it prepares her for regulating them later when seeing the entire word, a visualised spider or a real one.

Embedded suggestions:

- You know[FV] with the laser... *you can write with a laser.*
- Hmm[DM] I want you to[ER] *see it write the letter S on the cloud.*
- What I'd like you also to do[ER] *with your mind*, you know[DM], what you can *do with your mind is* you can[MO] *switch that laser off.*
- And[DM] you just have to[MO], *with your mind*, you just have to[MO] *say "off".*
- There *it goes on again.*

Direct suggestions:

- *You watch her looking up at the cloud write the letter S.*

Dependent suggestions:

- WHEN you *say "off" - that laser will go off.*

Adjunctive suggestions:

- So *stay back here* - AND *look at her lying on the beach.*
- Just *think it to yourself in your mind* now - AND *watch the laser goes off.*
- Now *say "on"* - AND *watch it go on again.*

Questions with an embedded suggestion:

- You *see that letter S appear on the cloud?*

Direct statement:

- There *it goes on again.*

Vague language:

- Vague verb: stay, switch on/off

- Unspecified place: back here, there
- Unspecified object/event: it
- Permissive: you can

Presuppositions:

- Repetitive cue word:
  what I'd like you also to do ⊇ you already do something
  watch it go on again ⊇ it was on before

- Pseudo-cleft sentence:
  what I'd like you also to do ⊇ I'd like you to do something
  what you can do with your mind is... ⊇ you can do something with your mind

Implications:

- have you ever seen that done ⊃ it has been done
- you just have to say "off" ⊃ saying "off" is easy and effective

Various techniques:

- Ratifying nonverbal response: "that's it"
- Checking her experience: "have you done that? "
- Dissociation: "look at *her* lying on the beach"; "*watch* the laser goes off"
- Metaphor: 'controlling the laser' stands for 'regulating her feelings'

Client: Yeah.

Brooks: So now, *you see the letter S up there* (pointing upwards). I want you to *allow the ... allow the laser to write ... the letter P.* (making writing movement in the air). (5 sec.) Do you *feel okay about watching it write like this*?

Client: Yeah.

Brooks: Yeah, okay. Just *notice how you feel* AS *you stay back here, looking at her look at the laser* (pointing at the three different locations for 'you', 'her' and 'the laser'). Now you can *write ... the letter I. Let it write the word.* You know what the word is, do you not? S, P, I ... (gesturing up as if writing the letters in the air).

Client: Spider.

Brooks: Spider. *Let her write the whole word.* And *you just stay here watching her on the beach looking up at that cloud.* You're not her, *you're just watching her.* And *we're going to help her do this.* (8 sec.) Let me know when *it has written the whole word.*

Step by step, Brooks has her visualise the letters of the word SPIDER. Note that he leaves a brief pause before he says: "The letter P". If she knows what letter is coming, she can already see it before it is mentioned; this means she is doing well. If she doesn't know, the pause will build up expectation, and she will be relieved to hear the letter when it finally comes. The same pause occurs before the next letter, 'I'. Brooks' pronunciation of the letter/word 'I' is ambiguous. The client will consciously interpret it as the third letter of the word SPIDER, but unconsciously she might interpret it as 'I as a person' and assert herself this way. Only after she has created the letters P and I, does Brooks go for the entire word. Rather than saying it he hints at it: "You know what word that is." Now, this can be a statement or a suggestion, depending on whether she already knew the word or only knows it now; perhaps it is a little of both. In Ericksonian hypnotherapy, the lines are blurred between the three sentence types statements, questions and commands. Questions and statements often act as commands (suggestions). Statements or suggestions are often intended to elicit or provoke information, so they act like questions. So Brooks hints at the word SPIDER, waits until she says it, and then suggests that she see it. Now, she has created an auditory and visual experience of the word SPIDER, but her feelings are dissociated. Brooks makes sure she stays in the double dissociation ("You're not her, you're just watching her"). Her body language shows no signs of fear or distress.

Embedded suggestions:

- So[DM] now[TA] *you see the letter S up there.*
- I want you to[ER] *allow the laser to write the letter P.*
- Now[TA] you can[MO] *write the letter I.*
- And[DM] you just[DA] *stay here watching her on the beach looking up at that cloud.*

- And[DM] *we're going to help her do this.*

Direct suggestions:

- *Let it write the word.*
- *Let her write the whole word.*

Dependent suggestions:

- Just *notice how you feel* - AS *you stay back here, looking at her look at the laser.*

Questions with an embedded suggestion:

- Do you *feel okay about watching it write like this*?

Instructions with an embedded suggestion:

- Let me know when *it has written the whole word.*

Embedded statement:

- You know what the word is, do you not[TQ]?

Direct statement:

- You're not her, you're *just watching her.*

Vague language:

- Vague verb: help
- Unspecified person: we
- Unspecified object/event: this, the word
- Definite article: *the* word (suggestion of specificity)
- Mind reading: you know what the word is
- Permissive: you can

Presuppositions:

- Noun clause:
  just notice how you feel $\supseteq$ you feel in a certain way
- Subordinate clause of time:
  let me know when it has written the whole word $\supseteq$ it will write the whole word

- Change-of-place verb:
  as you <u>stay</u> back here ⊇ you are back here now
  you just <u>stay</u> here ⊇ you are here now

- Gerund phrase:
  do you feel okay about <u>watching it write like this</u>? ⊇ you are watching it write like this

Various techniques:

- Checking her experience: "do you feel okay about watching it write like this? "
- Dissociation: implicitly: "*let her* write the whole word"; explicitly: "*you're not her, you're just watching her*"
- Hypnotic desensitisation: having her visualise the word spider before the image of it

Client: Yeah.

Brooks: Okay? How do you feel looking up at that word? *You feel okay*, do you not?

It is important that she can feel comfortable looking at the word before she goes to the next step. Brooks is checking 'if' she feels okay and at the same time suggesting 'that' she feels okay. As we saw before, the line between asking and suggesting is a fine one. The tag question ("do you not?") discharges any conscious doubt about feeling okay.

Client: Yeah.

Brooks: *It's okay, no problem at all.*

Client: No (shakes her head).

Client: (eyelids flutter once) Mmm.

Brooks: Okay, what I'd like you to do is *watch the cloud* kind of *get misty, a little bit misty* AND *absorb those ... letters into the cloud* (pointing upwards, moving his fingers), SO *the word becomes absorbed into the cloud.* Let me know when *it's just faded away into the cloud.*

Client: Mmm.

Brooks: Okay, faded away into the clouds now? Yes?

Client: Yeah.

Making the letters of the word 'spider' disappear into the cloud is a metaphor for her ability to make her fear disappear. It is a way of seeding problem resolution. Furthermore, is a good test: if she follows the suggestion of making the word disappear, she is unconsciously agreeing to make her problem disappear. Conversely, if she has reasons to keep her fear, she will probably have difficulty making the word disappear. This section is also a good example of the art of repetition. Brooks repeats the idea of absorption with a five-step suggestion:

- what I'd like you to do is *watch the cloud kind of get misty*
- and *absorb those letters into the cloud*
- so *the word becomes absorbed into the cloud*
- let me know when *it's just faded away into the cloud.*
- *faded away in the cloud* now?

Within these five steps, he uses an embedded suggestion (what I'd like you to do is), linking (and, so), an implication (let me know when…) and a question (faded away…?).

Embedded suggestions:

- *You feel okay* do you not[TQ]?
- Okay[DM] what I'd like you to[ER] do is *watch the cloud* kind of[LS] *get misty.*

Adjunctive suggestion and cause-effect link:

- *Watch the cloud* kind of *get misty* - AND *absorb those letters into the cloud* - SO *the word becomes absorbed into the cloud.*

Instructions with an embedded suggestion:

- Let me know when *it's just faded away into the cloud.*

Direct suggestions:

- *It's okay, no problem at all.*

Vague language:

- Nominalisation: problem
- Vague verb: absorbed, faded
- Unspecified object/event: it
- Mind reading: you feel okay

Presuppositions:

- Subordinate clause of time:
  let me know when it's just faded away ⊇ it will fade away
- Qualifying adverb:
  no problem at all ⊇ no problem
  a little bit misty ⊇ a bit misty ⊇ misty
  when it's just faded away ⊇ when it's faded away
- Demonstrative determiner:
  that word ⊇ there is a specific word
- Pseudo-cleft sentence:
  what I'd like you to do is ⊇ I'd like you to do something
- Gerund phrase:
  How do you feel looking up at that word? ⊇ you are looking up at that word

Various techniques:

- Metaphor: 'making the word spider disappear' stands for 'making her fear disappear'

Brooks: Okay. What I want to do, in a moment I'm going to touch you on the right-hand shoulder like this (touches her briefly on her right shoulder). Okay? I'm going to touch you on the right shoulder like this (touches the right shoulder again). I'd like you to notice that you can *go veeery, veeery deeply* ***relaxed***. And you'll know *that can happen* BECAUSE *your whole body become, can become,* ***lovely*** *and* ***relaxed***. Do you know about these rag dolls?

After the exercise in dissociation and making something disappear, Brooks starts another 'deepening' phase. He creates a kinaesthetic anchor for relaxation by touching her on the shoulder. He does this in his typical way, which is different from the standard NLP way of anchoring. He announces that he will touch her on the shoulder and briefly touches her. This way, her conscious mind knows what's coming but has no time to really think or worry about it. She can immediately feel how it is and feel if it is okay. So, Brooks communicates on two levels here: verbally and nonverbally. Both her verbal and nonverbal reactions are positive. Brooks then suggests more relaxation. Let's look at his suggestion, "I'd like you to notice that you can *go veeery, veeery deeply relaxed*", and how it differs from the simple, direct suggestion "relax deeply". This suggestion is:

> Threefold indirect: I'd like you to notice that you can *go very, very deeply relaxed*
>
> Twofold implicative: 'very deeply relaxed' presupposes 'deeply relaxed' which presupposes 'relaxed'
>
> Dramatic: by repeating and stretching out the word *veeery*

The next sentence is: "And you'll know that can happen because your whole body become, can become, lovely and relaxed". On the one hand, this is simply a way of repeating the same idea (relaxation). On the other hand, it is another way of depotentiating the conscious mind. The conscious mind wants to know and logically understand what happens. Brooks here satisfies both needs by saying, "You'll *know* that can happen *because...*" The unconscious does not need logical explanations and will simply follow the suggestion of relaxation. Relaxation is then further enhanced with the metaphor of a rag doll.

Embedded suggestions:

- I'd like you to[ER] notice[FV] that you can[MO] *go very, very deeply relaxed.*

Adjunctive suggestion:

- And you'll know *that can happen* - BECAUSE *your whole body can become lovely and relaxed.*

Embedded statement:

- <u>In a moment</u>[TA], I'm going to touch you on the right-hand shoulder like this.

Direct statement:

- I'm going to touch you on the right shoulder like this.

Vague language:

- Vague verb: go relaxed, happen
- Vague adjective: relaxed, lovely
- Ambiguous (homonym): *right* shoulder
- Permissive: you can

Presuppositions:

- Qualifying adverb:
  <u>very</u> <u>deeply</u> relaxed ⊇ <u>deeply</u> relaxed ⊇ relaxed

- Pseudo-cleft sentence:
  <u>what</u> I want to do... ⊇ I want to do something

Client: Mmm.

Brooks: You know? Ready? So, on the count of three, on the count of three, I'll touch you on the shoulder AND just *let aaall the muscles just become looose and relaxed.* One, two, three (puts his hand on her shoulder), just *relax every muscle*, thaaat's it, *aaall the way down*, that's it. You're doing very, very well. Just *relax eeevery muscle ... eevery muscle.* ... ANYTIME I touch you on the shoulder here (briefly releases his hand and touches her shoulder again), you can just *relax all the way, all the way like this, nice and relaxed, and comfortable.* ANYTIME you feel me touch you on the shoulder here (briefly releasing and retouching her shoulder) *your whole body can just become soooo comfortable relaxed, so comfortable relaxed, very relaxed and comfortable, deeeeper relaxed.* You're doing very well ... very well (releases his hand from her shoulder).

> Here Brooks actually sets (creates) the kinaesthetic anchor he announced and initiated before. First, he asks her if she is ready. He knows she is ready but answering this question enhances the yes-set and brings the

process further under her control. Counting to three builds up expectation, and it might also trigger childhood experiences of surprise or excitement. After all the announcing, demonstrating, asking and counting, she is now more than ready to receive the touch on the shoulder, and the relaxation that it is suggested will come with that. Once an anchor (in this case a touch) is set, it can be repeated later, and it will elicit the corresponding state (in this case relaxation). Brooks reinforces this natural response by suggesting it: "Anytime I touch you on the shoulder here, you can just relax all the way." When he repeats this suggestion, it is slightly different: "Any time *you feel* me touch you on the shoulder." A typical shift from external experience (him doing something) to internal experience (her feeling something). Nonverbal support for relaxation is not just in the touch, it's also in his voice; some words are stretched out and some are just whispered. Finally, in this section, he compliments her again for her inner work.

Embedded suggestions:

- Just[DA] *relax every muscle*, that's it, *all the way down.*
- You can[MO] just[DA] *relax all the way like this, nice and relaxed, and comfortable.*

Dependent suggestions:

- ANYTIME I touch you on the shoulder here - you can just *relax all the way like this.*
- ANYTIME you feel me touch you on the shoulder here - *your whole body can just become so comfortable, relaxed.*

Adjunctive suggestions:

- I'll touch you on the shoulder - AND just *let all the muscles just become loose and relaxed.*

Vague language:

- Nominalisation: count
- Vague verb: become loose, relax
- Vague adjective: ready, loose, relaxed, nice, comfortable
- Unspecified object/event: this

- Unspecified process: like this
- Universal quantifier: every muscle, anytime
- Permissive: you can

Presuppositions:

- Subordinate clause of time:
  anytime I touch you on the shoulder $\supseteq$ I will touch you on the shoulder

- Qualifying adverb:
  let all the muscles just become loose $\supseteq$ let all the muscles become loose
  all the way down $\supseteq$ down
  so comfortable relaxed $\supseteq$ comfortable relaxed $\supseteq$ relaxed
  very relaxed $\supseteq$ relaxed

Implications:

- Ready? One, two, three... $\supset$ something important is about to happen

Various techniques:

- Complimenting: "you're doing very well"
- Ratifying nonverbal response: "that's it"

Brooks: (leaning back and changing his voice to more firm intonation) Now *look at her on the beach* (pointing to a place in front of her). *She is still lying there looking at the cloud.* And together now, the two of us (pointing at the client and himself), *we are going to help her.* The next step *we're gonna help her* ... Because there are a number of steps (indicating imaginary steps in the air) in what *we're going to do for her,* and that's the first step ... she has just achieved, SO she's done very well. So, I'd like to *congratulate her.* Maybe you want to *congratulate her for doing the first step.* You can *do that to yourself, in your mind.* (5 sec.)

After the deepening phase, Brooks introduces the idea of a number of steps to be taken. Splitting the process into several steps —and congratulating her for having taken the first one— makes it easy for her to follow. Breaking a problem into manageable pieces is a general technique that Brooks uses. It is also a way of utilising part of her thinking style: following procedures. Brooks is also further developing the idea of the two of them working as a team to help her. Note the two-step congratulation, shifting from external to internal. First "I congratulate her" then "You can congratulate her". Brooks is planting more seeds for the client to take responsibility for her own healing and change.

Embedded suggestions:

- Now[DM] *look at her on the beach.*
- Maybe[SA] you want to[MO] *congratulate her for doing the first step.*
- You can[MO] *do that to yourself in your mind.*

Cause-effect link:

- That's the first step she has just achieved - SO she's done very well.

Direct suggestions:

- *She is still lying there looking at the cloud.*

Embedded statements:

- And[DM] together now[TA] the two of us, *we are going to help her.*
- Because[DM] there are a number of steps in what *we're going to do for her.*
- So[DM], I'd like to[MO] *congratulate her.*

Direct statements:

- The next step *we're gonna help her.*

Vague language:

- Nominalisation: step
- Vague verb: help, achieve, congratulate
- Unspecified quantity: a number of
- No pronoun subject: *there are* a number of steps
- Permissive: maybe, you can
- Mind reading: she is still lying there looking at the cloud

Presuppositions:

- Ordinal numeral:
  the next step ⊇ there have been other steps
  the first step ⊇ there will be more steps

- Change-of-time adverb:
  she is still lying there ⊇ she has been lying there for a while

- Noun clause:
  in what we're going to do for her ⊇ we're going to do something for her

- Qualifying adverb:
  she's done very well ⊇ she's done well
  she has just achieved ⊇ she has achieved

Various techniques:

- Dissociation: "you can do that *to yourself*"; "*she* has just achieved"; "maybe you want to congratulate *her*"
- Enhancing cooperation: "together"; "the two of us"

Brooks: You know *these lasers, they can project images and pictures* as well (pointing upwards), s*till pictures, moving pictures*. The first thing that *it is going to project is a still picture* ... , BUT *it's gonna be difficult to see what it is*. So just *switch the laser on* now, you know how to do that. *Set it on*, AND WHEN *it projects up*, *you watch her*. Because *she's gonna see an image or a picture appear on the cloud*, BUT *she can't make out what it is at first, on the cloud* ... (puts his hand on her shoulder). Just *get her to see that* now (releases his hand). And AS that *image or picture starts to form* ... I want you to *watch her* ... Because *she's gonna be very relaxed on the beach*, *totally relaxed and confident and comfortable* (gesturing in front of her). *You watch her*. Because *she's gonna see that image and that picture* (pointing up) *start to take shape*. And *it's gonna become ... a picture of that word that she saw up there* AND *she's gonna* **feel veeery comfortable**. And just *watch her now* **feel very comfortable** (touching her on the shoulder). If you think at any time she could feel uncomfortable, just *say the word 'off'* (releasing his hand) AND *the laser will switch itself off* ... And then *switch it on again and watch it again* (touching her on the shoulder) ... You might even want to ... (releasing his hand) *try switching it on and off a few times* (briefly touching her on the shoulder). Just so you can notice that ... ***you can do that***, AND that she can ***feel totally comfortable*** *looking at that picture ... on that cloud, up there*. Just *watch her now*.

After seeing —and then hiding— the word SPIDER, and further relaxation and deepening, it is now time for the next step: seeing the 'image' of a spider. Again, Brooks does this in a gradual, stepwise way, making sure that the client stays in a state of comfort and control. First, he gives her an illusionary choice: a still picture or a moving picture. Whatever she chooses, she will see a picture; this is, therefore, a double bind. Immediately, he limits her choice by telling her to see a still picture first. This, of course, implies that she will see a moving picture later. Her conscious mind can look at the relatively 'safe' still picture while her unconscious can prepare for a moving picture. Any possible reluctance or unwillingness to see a spider is anticipated by suggesting that the image will be 'difficult to see'. This technique is called 'prescribing' a problem. It normalises the problem before it arises and brings it under the hypnotherapist's control. If the client has difficulty seeing it, it now means she is cooperating. She can feel fine about it and rapport is maintained (yes-set). If she has no difficulty seeing it, she is doing better than predicted and can feel proud of this. Now look at the stepwise serial suggestions Brooks uses here:

- it's gonna be difficult to see what it is: prescribing possible difficulty
- she can't make out what it is at first: prescribing difficulty but implying she can see it later
- as that image or picture starts to form: suggesting that she *starts to* see an *undefined* picture
- it's gonna become a picture of that word: suggesting a *defined* picture of a *spider*

During this procedure, he makes sure she maintains her state of dissociation, comfort and control by careful observation, suggestion and anchoring. At this point, she has made a major step forward in solving her problem: she can now think about a spider and feel comfortable.

This is in stark contrast to her response at the beginning of the session, a mere twenty minutes earlier.

Embedded suggestions:

- You know[DM] *these lasers they can project images and pictures* as well, s*till pictures, moving pictures.*
- So[DM] just[DA] *switch the laser on* now[TA].
- Just[DA] *get her to see that* now[TA].
- Because[DM] *she's gonna be very relaxed on the beach, totally relaxed and confident and comfortable.*
- Because[DM] *she's gonna see that image and that picture start to take shape.*
- And[DM] just[DA] *watch her* now[TA] *feel very comfortable.*
- And[DM] then[TA] *switch it on again and watch it again.*
- You might[MO] even want to[MO] *try switching it on and off a few times.*
- Just[DA] so you can[MO] notice[FV] that *you can do that.*
- She can[MO] *feel totally comfortable looking at that picture.*
- Just[DA] *watch her now.*

Direct suggestions:

- *You watch her.*

Dependent suggestions:

- AS *that image or picture starts to form* - I want you to *watch her.*

Adjunctive suggestions:

- The first thing that *it is going to project is a still picture* - BUT *it's gonna be difficult to see what it is.*
- *She's gonna see an image or a picture appear on the cloud* - BUT *she can't make out what it is at first.*
- *It's gonna become a picture of that word that she saw up there* - AND *she's gonna feel very comfortable.*
- Then *switch it on again* - AND *watch it again.*
- Just *say the word 'off'* - AND *the laser will switch itself off.*

- You can notice that *you can do that* - AND that *she can feel totally comfortable.*

Dependent/adjunctive suggestions:

- *Set it on* - AND - WHEN *it projects up - you watch her.*

Vague language:

- Nominalisation: shape
- Vague adjective: relaxed, difficult, confident, comfortable, important, integral
- Vague adverb: totally, automatically, easily
- Unspecified time: at any time
- Unspecified place: up there
- Unspecified object/event: these lasers, that
- Unspecified frequency: a few times
- No personal pronoun (infinitive): it's gonna be difficult to see what it is
- Permissive: you might, you can
- Mind reading: you know how to do that

Presuppositions:

- Relative clause:
  the first thing <u>that</u> it is going to project ⊇ it is going to project a thing
  that word <u>that</u> she saw ⊇ she saw that word

- Ordinal numeral:
  <u>the first thing</u> that it is going to project... ⊇ it will project more things

- Subordinate clause of time:
  <u>when</u> it projects up ⊇ it will project up

- Repetitive cue word:

they can project images and pictures <u>as well</u> ⊇ they already projected other things (referring to the letters of the word SPIDER)

switch it on <u>again</u> ⊇ you switched it on before

watch it <u>again</u> ⊇ you watched it before

- Qualifying adverb:

  she's gonna feel <u>very</u> comfortable ⊇ she's gonna feel comfortable

  she can feel <u>totally</u> comfortable ⊇ she can feel comfortable

  you might <u>even</u> want to ⊇ you might want to

  be <u>very</u> relaxed ⊇ be relaxed

- Demonstrative determiner:

  she's gonna see <u>that</u> image ⊇ there is a specific image

  a picture of <u>that</u> word ⊇ there is a specific word (referring to the word SPIDER)

Implications:

- she can't make out what it is <u>at first</u> ⊃ she will make out what it is later

Various techniques:

- Suggesting automatic processes: "laser will switch *itself* off"

Brooks: And you might like to *notice the fluttering in your eyelids* at this moment. I told you how that would *help you with this* ... Because THE MORE *your eyelids flutter* ... AS *you go through this*, *THE EASIER it's gonna be* ... to *allow this to happen ... automatically, easily and* ***comfortably***. And you might wonder how you knew or how a part of you knew, that *your eyelids had to flutter to help you experience this.* That flutter in your eyelids is an important, integral part ... of ***making these changes happen***. And you *discover that,* AS you go along.

Brooks observes her eyelids fluttering again and utilises this to ratify links he created earlier in the session:

eyelids fluttering → trance → therapeutic change

The fact that she has changed so much already and that her eyelids are fluttering again ‘proves’ this connection. Obviously, this is not scientific proof, but it is created by suggestion. It is like saying to someone, “You are thinking about a red balloon now”. By the time you say the word ‘now‘, the listener is very likely to think about a red balloon. He or she has to, in order to understand what you are saying. This is, in a sense, a created reality. Brooks earlier ‘told’ her unconscious mind, “If you make your eyelids flutter, I see that as a sign of trance and therapeutic change”. Look at the suggestion “You might wonder how you knew, or how a part of you knew, that your eyelids had to flutter to help you experience this”. It is an indirect compliment to the unconscious for picking up on the earlier suggestion. For the conscious mind, ‘proving’ his earlier statement about this connection increases his authority and thereby her conscious belief that he can help her. Brooks defines fluttering as an integral part of change. He tells her conscious mind that it will discover this while suggesting to her unconscious to make more changes happen, and to show these changes by fluttering the eyelids.

Embedded suggestions:

- And[DM] you might[MO] like to[MO] *notice the fluttering in your eyelids* at this moment[TA].

Dependent suggestions:

- You *discover that* - AS you go along.

Correlative comparative and dependent suggestion:

- THE MORE *your eyelids flutter* - AS *you go through this* - *THE EASIER it's gonna be* to *allow this to happen automatically*, *easily and comfortably*.

Embedded statements:

- And[DM] you might[MO] wonder[EQ] how you knew, or how a part of you knew, that *your eyelids had to flutter to help you experience this.*

Direct statements:

- I told you how that would *help you with this.*

- That flutter in your eyelids is an important, integral part of *making these changes happen.*

Vague language:

- Nominalisation: changes
- Vague verb: help, wonder, experience, making...happen, discover
- Vague adjective: easy, important, integral
- Vague adverb: automatically, easily, comfortably
- Unspecified object/event: that
- Permissive: you might
- Mind reading: you might wonder

Presuppositions:

- Subordinate clause of time:
  as you go through this $\supseteq$ you go through this
- Embedded question:
  you might wonder how you knew $\supseteq$ you knew
- Demonstrative determiner:
  that flutter $\supseteq$ there is a specific flutter

Implications:

- the fluttering in your eyelids at this moment $\supset$ the fluttering may change or stop later

Various techniques:

- Conscious/unconscious dissociation: "how a *part of you* knew..."
- Validating the unconscious: "part of you *knew*"

Brooks: Okay, so can she see the picture up there now?

Client: Yeah.

Brooks: And how do you feel about her watching it?

Client: Fine.

Brooks: You feel fine. And she looks *comfortable down on the beach*? (pointing to a place in front of her)

Client: Yeah.

Brooks: Okay, so *she feels okay about it* as well?

Client: Yeah.

> Brooks is asking a few questions to check her state of dissociation and comfort as well as enhance those states. She is looking at herself, looking at the cloud and feels fine. This is important if she is to continue the process of desensitisation.
>
> Questions with an embedded suggestion:
>
> - Can she *see the picture up there* now?
> - And *she looks comfortable down on the beach*?
> - So *she feels okay about it* as well?
>
> Presuppositions:
>
> - Question:
>   <u>how</u> do you feel about her watching it? ⊇ you feel something about her watching it
>
> - Repetitive cue word:
>   she feels okay about it <u>as well</u> ⊇ someone else (her dissociated self) already feels okay about it
>
> - Gerund phrase:
>   How do you feel about <u>her watching it</u>? ⊇ she is watching it
>
> Various techniques:
>
> - Checking the client's experience: "how do you feel about…?"

Brooks: Okay, that's fine. Now you know you can still *control the laser anytime you want*. You can *say "on" or "off", anytime you want*. What I would like you to do, you know, is ***you have control*** *over the cloud* as well. You can *move it around the sky* (using a high-pitched voice). How about moving it over ... over this side (pointing to her right, directing his voice to her right), over here? Can you *move* *it over here*? And *let her ... let her watch it* AS *it moves over this side.* Let's *move it over here, over this side in the sky.* (5 sec.) So now *move it back again ... over there* (pointing to her left side), *over there, move it back over there.* That's it. You're doing very well. A very good job. I'd like you to *move it up, push it up* (making a pushing up movement, using a high-pitched voice), *make it go higher up, do that* as well. Notice *the picture gets a bit smaller.* Then *stop it,* BEFORE it goes too far. Then *bring it back again, back down again* (making a downward gesture), *to where it was.* (14 sec.) Now you can *bring it lower, bring it down lower ...* SO *it gets a little bit bigger ... a little bit closer.* And *bring it as low* (using a low-pitched voice) *as you can ... as low as it feels comfortable.* You're gonna *bring the cloud all the way down to the ground or to the sea.* You can *do that* if you want ... SO *it's comfortable.* Only as low as *it feels comfortable for you.* (16 sec.)

The next step is bringing the picture down, closer to the version of herself on the beach. Again, Brooks does this stepwise, utilising her thinking style. First, he has her move the cloud around to increase her sense of control even further. Then he uses the typical Ericksonian technique of going the opposite way first, in this case moving the picture up. This is probably easier for her than bringing it down; at the same time, it proves that she can control its proximity. Only then does he instruct her to move it down and bring it closer. Nonverbally he helps her to lower the picture by lowering his voice. Note the sentence "...*bring it as low as you can, as low as it feels comfortable*". It challenges her (as low as you can) and at the same time protects her (as low as feels comfortable). Also, challenging someone to do a difficult task and then making it a little simpler is a technique used to make the task acceptable for the client. Brooks repeats the same technique with the challenging task 'all the way down' followed by the easier one 'only as low as it feels comfortable'. Furthermore, bringing the cloud down is linked to comfort, first implicitly (as low as feels comfortable), then explicitly (bring the cloud all the way down...so it feels comfortable).

Embedded suggestions:

- Now[DM] you know[FV] you can[MO] still *control the laser anytime you want.*
- You can[MO] *say "on" or "off" anytime you want.*
- What I would like you to[ER] do you know[DM], is *you have control over the cloud.*

- You can[MO] *move it around the sky.*
- Let's *move it over here, over this side in the sky.*
- So[DM] now[TA] *move it back again, over there.*
- I'd like you to[ER] *move it up, push it up.*
- Notice[FV] *the picture gets a bit smaller.*
- Then[TA] *bring it back again, back down again to where it was.*
- And[DM] *bring it as low as you can, as low as it feels comfortable.*
- You're gonna[A] *bring the cloud all the way down to the ground or to the sea.*

Questions with an embedded suggestion:

- Can you *move it over here?*

Dependent suggestions:

- And *let her watch it* - AS *it moves over this side.*
- Then *stop it* - BEFORE it goes too far.

Cause-effect link:

- Now you can *bring it down lower* - SO *it gets a little bit bigger.*
- You can *do that* if you want - SO *it's comfortable.*

Vague language:

- Nominalisation: control, job
- Vague adjective: fine, comfortable
- Unspecified place: around the sky, this side, in the sky, over there, up, too far, lower, all the way down
- Unspecified object/event: it, that's fine
- Comparative deletion: smaller, lower, bigger, closer
- Permissive: you can

Presuppositions:

- Pseudo-cleft sentence:
  what I would like you to do you know is... ⊇ I would like you to do something

- Subordinate clause of time:
  before it goes too far ⊇ it could go too far
- Change-of-time adverb:
  you can still control the laser ⊇ you could control the laser before
- Repetitive cues word:
  move it back over there ⊇ it was over there before
  bring it back again⊇ it was there before
  do that as well ⊇ you did other things
- Qualifying adverb:
  picture gets a bit smaller ⊇ picture gets smaller
  a little bit closer ⊇ closer

Implications:

- only as low as it feels comfortable for you ⊃ it could go lower

Various techniques:

- Ratifying nonverbal response: "okay"; "that's fine"; "that's it"
- Complimenting: "you're doing very well"; "a very good job"
- Opposite direction: "I'd like you to *move it up*"

Brooks: (touches her on the shoulder) Okay, *deep for you to* ***feel relaxed and comfortable*** (releases his touch). Now, that picture ... how low is it, how low is that cloud at the moment (making a downward gesture)? Is it on the ground yet, or is it still up in the air?

Client: On the horizon.

Brooks: On the horizon? Well done. Doing very, very well, have it on the horizon. Now *keeping it on the horizon* (gesturing towards the distance), what I want you to do, is *ask her* (pointing in front of her) *to look at it* on the horizon. In your mind *ask her to look at it*, AND to *bring it forward towards her* (gesturing towards her) ... *comfortably* ... SO *it's closer* ... BUT only *as close as it's comfortable for her.* Just to see how *close ... she can bring it.* Just *get her to do that*, AS *you watch.* (5 sec.) (Touching her on the shoulder and switching to a softer voice) Just ***feel***

comfortable and relaxed, even *deeper relaxed ... deeper and deeper relaxed* (15 sec.)(letting go of her shoulder).

The client has brought the picture *down*, but not *closer* to herself as Brooks suggested. Nevertheless, he compliments her. This is an important principle; to accept, appreciate and utilise any response from your client. Every response is interpreted as cooperation. It is a bit like your car's satellite navigation system: if you ignore an instruction and take a 'wrong' turn, it does not criticise you; it simply recalculates the route from your current position and tells you what to do next. Similarly, an Ericksonian hypnotherapist constantly re-evaluates his next step based on the client's response to the previous step. Brooks talks about 'flying by the seat of your pants' in this respect. Here, he compliments the client for putting the picture on the horizon. Telling her to keep it there further implies that putting it there was okay. Only then does he suggest that she begin bringing it closer, again using her state of dissociation (ask *her* to...) and relaxation (touching her on her shoulder). Let's have a look at the suggestion 'only as close as it's comfortable for her, just to see how close she can bring it'. This is a nice example of multi-level communication. The conscious mind gets two *explicit* suggestions: 'observe what happens and make sure it does not get too close'. The unconscious mind is challenged with two *implied* suggestions: 'bring it as close as you can and be comfortable'. The idea is that the unconscious 'wins' and the conscious mind can experience that a 'close' picture of a spider is nothing to fear. The general idea is to reassure, distract or confuse the conscious mind so that the unconscious can create something new and the conscious mind can then experience that that is okay. As he did in all previous steps, Brooks helps the client to take this step with suggestions of comfort and relaxation.

Embedded suggestions:

- Okay[DM] *deep for you to feel relaxed and comfortable.*
- Now[DM] *keeping it on the horizon.*
- What I want you to[ER] do, is *ask her to look at it on the horizon.*
- Just[DA] to *see how close she can bring it.*

- Just[DA] *feel comfortable and relaxed,* even *deeper relaxed.*

Dependent suggestions:

- Just *get her to do that* - AS *you watch.*

Adjunctive suggestions and cause-effect link:

- *Ask her to look at it on the horizon* - AND *bring it forward towards her comfortably* - SO *it's closer* - BUT only *as close as it's comfortable for her.*

Vague language:

- Nominalisation: horizon
- Vague adjective: relaxed, deep
- Vague adverb: comfortably
- Unspecified time: at the moment
- Unspecified place: on the horizon
- Comparative deletion: deeper
- No personal pronoun (gerund): *doing* very, very well

Presuppositions:

- Question:
  how low is that cloud? $\supseteq$ that cloud is low

- Change-of-time adverb:
  is it on the ground yet? $\supseteq$ it will be on the ground
  is it still up in the air? $\supseteq$ it will not stay up in the air

- Qualifying adverb:
  even deeper relaxed $\supseteq$ deeper relaxed $\supseteq$ relaxed

- Demonstrative determiner:
  that cloud $\supseteq$ there is a specific cloud
  that picture $\supseteq$ there is a specific picture

- Pseudo-cleft sentence:
  what I want you to do is... $\supseteq$ I want you to do something

Implications:

- how low is that cloud <u>at the moment</u> ⊃ it could – or will - be lower later
- is it <u>still</u> up in the air ⊃ it will not remain up in the air

Various techniques:

- Complimenting: "well done"; "doing very very well"
- Frustrating response: "but *only as close* as it's comfortable for her"

Brooks: How *close is it now*?

Client: Quite near.

Brooks: Quite near. And how do you feel looking at her, looking at that?

Client: Fine.

Brooks: Fine. How does she feel?

Client: Fine.

Brooks: Fine, okay. (8 sec.) Okay, well *thank her for doing that.* That's the next step. *Thank her for doing that for you.* And she's gonna thank you later, for *helping her achieve this* as well.

The client has been able to bring the picture of the spider closer now and feels fine with that. Brooks lets one part (the double dissociated self) of her thank the other part (the single dissociated self), which enforces her state of dissociation. He predicts that the other part will return the thanks later. Whether this will happen or not does not matter; the idea enhances the state of gratitude and brings her current experience —of feeling comfortable while looking at a close picture of a spider— into the future. The prediction also implies that something positive will be achieved: something to be grateful for. The phrase 'for helping her achieve this as well' is an ambiguity of scope. The phrase 'as well' can refer to 'helping her and thereby imply 'she also helped you', or it can refer to 'achieve this' and imply 'she achieved other things'.

Embedded suggestions:

- <u>Okay</u>^{DM}, <u>well</u>^{DM} *thank her for doing that.*

Direct suggestion:

- *Thank her for doing that for you.*

Embedded statement:

- <u>And</u>[DM] she's gonna thank you later, for *helping her achieve this* as well.

Direct statement:

- That's the next step.

Vague language:

- Vague verb: helping, achieve
- Unspecified place: close, near
- Unspecified object/event: that, this
- Ambiguity (of scope): as well

Presuppositions:

- Question:
  <u>how</u> close is it now? ⊇ it is close

- Repetitive cue word:
  that's the <u>next</u> step ⊇ there have been previous steps
  for helping her achieve this <u>as well</u> ⊇ you helped her achieve other things

- Gerund phrase:
  how do you feel <u>looking at her</u> ⊇ you are looking at her

Various techniques:

- Dissociation: "how do you feel *looking at her, looking at that?*"

Brooks: Now, I'd like you to ... *find* ... *somewhere convenient* ... *to rest that cloud, somewhere on the ground, somewhere.* Just *rest the cloud, somewhere, somewhere convenient, not too far away* ... *nearby.* (Touches her on the shoulder, switches to softer voice) Just ***feel comfortable and relaxed***, AS *you allow that to happen.* (He lets go of her shoulder after 8 seconds.)(12 sec.) And AS *you watch her now* ... *nearby* ... *that cloud, with that picture of it* ... *you have the laser still on that cloud*, EVEN THOUGH *it's now* *down by the ground.* **You can switch it off**, if you want. *You can switch it on, it's up to you.*

Bringing the picture of the spider closer has probably been a challenging step for her. It means confronting herself with her biggest fear. Brooks takes the time to congratulate her, support her and help her feel comfortable, relaxed and in control. Just look at the first sentence here: "Now, I'd like you to find somewhere convenient to rest that cloud." To her conscious mind, he is saying "Put that cloud somewhere and let it rest". To her unconscious, he says "Y*ou* can rest conveniently", using:

Embedded suggestion: Now, I'd like you to...

Implication: find somewhere convenient $\supseteq$ somewhere convenient exists

Unspecified place: somewhere

Metaphor: 'rest the cloud' stands for 'you can rest'

Then he brings back the idea of the laser to re-establish her sense of control over the picture, now that it is close to her.

Embedded suggestions:

- Now[DM], I'd like you to[ER] *find somewhere convenient to rest that cloud, somewhere on the ground.*
- Just[DA] *rest the cloud somewhere, somewhere convenient.*

Direct suggestions:

- *You can switch it off.*
- *You can switch it on, it's up to you.*

Dependent suggestions:

- Just *feel comfortable and relaxed* - AS *you allow that to happen.*

Dependent/adjunctive suggestion:

- AS *you watch her now.. - you have the laser still on that cloud* - EVEN THOUGH *it's now down by the ground.*

Vague language:

- Vague verb: rest
- Vague adjective: convenient, comfortable, relaxed
- Unspecified place: somewhere, not too far away, nearby, down by the ground
- Unspecified object/event: that, it
- Permissive: you can

Presuppositions:

- Change-of-time adverb:
  you have the laser still on that cloud $\supseteq$ the laser was already on the cloud

- Demonstrative determiner:
  that cloud/that picture $\supseteq$ there is a specific cloud/picture

Various techniques:

- Metaphor: 'rest that cloud' stands for 'her own state of rest'

Brooks: I'd like you to get it to move, get the picture to move a little bit. Stay on the cloud, BUT get it to move, that picture. Like a little home video or something. Just get it to move. (7 sec.) So you see that spider picture moving (touching her on the shoulder). Keep relaxed and comfortable, and relaxed (letting go of her shoulder). That's it. Doing very well. Can you see it moving now?

At this point in the session, it is time for the next step: seeing a *moving* spider on the cloud. Seeing a moving spider is bound to be more frightening for her, so Brooks re-establishes the anchor of relaxation and comfort.

Embedded suggestions:

- I'd like you[ER] to *get it to move, get the picture to move a little bit.*
- Just[DA] *get it to move.*
- So[DM] *you see that spider picture moving.*

Direct suggestion:

- *Keep relaxed and comfortable, and relaxed.*

Adjunctive suggestions:

- *Stay on the cloud* - BUT *get it to move, that picture.*

Questions with an embedded suggestion:

- Can you *see it moving* now?

Vague language:

- Vague adjective: relaxed, comfortable

Presuppositions:

- Change-of-time verb:
  stay on the cloud ⊇ you are on the cloud
  keep relaxed and comfortable ⊇ you are relaxed and comfortable

- Demonstrative determiner:
  that picture ⊇ there is a specific picture

Various techniques:

- Ratifying nonverbal response: "that's it"
- Small steps: "get the picture to move *a little bit*"

Client: Mmm.

Brooks: And how do you feel about watching her ... watching it move?

Client: Okay.

Brooks: It's okay. And how does she feel?

Client: Okay.

Brooks: Okay, as well. Good. Well *congratulate her on that.* That's the next step. Now, *notice how easy it has been, a step at a time.* They always say, you know, if *you take things a step at a time*, almost ***anything is possible***. *Notice how easy it has been, just taking things a step at a time.* (8 sec.)

Again, Brooks gives her a break from her challenging experience, inviting her to congratulate herself and acknowledge that another step has been taken. The process so far is defined as easy and connected to the goal of the session: overcoming her fear. Just look at the statement, "They always say, you know, if you take things a step at a time almost anything is possible". The message here is "Your problem can be solved". But it is stated vaguely and indirectly. Let's examine how Brooks turns a direct and specific suggestion into a vague and indirect one:

> your problem can be solved: a direct suggestion
>
> *anything is possible*: making it vague using a universal quantifier
>
> almost *anything is possible*: softening it and turning it into an implication
>
> if you take things a step at a time almost *anything is possible*: linking it the current process
>
> you know if you take things a step at a time almost *anything is possible*: making it indirect with a factive verb
>
> they always say you know if you take things a step at a time almost *anything is possible*: turning it into a quote

All these words are spoken in the space of a few seconds and, while her conscious mind is busy processing them, her unconscious mind can pick up the embedded message (*anything is possible*) and make it concrete (my problem can be solved). Furthermore, the suggestions of *anything being possible* and *it being easy* lie between two identical phrases 'a step at a time...a step at a time'. Repeating an earlier phrase enhances amnesia for the words in between. So, firstly, her conscious mind is distracted from the actual message, and then it is helped to forget it. Brooks doesn't have to consciously think about all this; he is unconsciously competent in Ericksonian language. The reader might want to practise this by creating various concrete and direct suggestions and then making them vague and indirect using any of the techniques described in this book.

Embedded suggestions:

- Well[DM] *congratulate her on that.*
- Now[DM] *notice how easy it has been a step at a time.*

- They always say[Q], you know[DM], if *you take things a step at a time* almost[LS] *anything is possible.*

Direct suggestions:

- *Notice how easy it has been, just taking things a step at a time.*

Direct statements:

- That's the next step.

Vague language:

- Nominalisation: step
- Vague adjective: easy
- Unspecified person: they
- Unspecified object/event: that, things
- Universal quantifier: always, anything
- Lost performant: if you take things a step at a time almost anything is possible
- No personal pronoun (gerund): notice how easy it has been taking things a step at a time

Presuppositions:

- Noun clause:
  notice how easy it has been ⊇ it has been easy

- Ordinal numeral:
  that's the next step ⊇ there have been steps already

- Repetitive cue word:
  okay as well ⊇ something else is okay

- Gerund phrase:
  how do you feel about watching her, watching it move ⊇ you are watching her, watching it move

Implications:

- congratulate her on 'that' ⊃ 'that' is valuable

Various techniques:

- Complimenting: "good! "
- Quote (unspecified source): "they always say... "

Brooks: Now, I want you to *do some dreaming, do a little bit of dreaming in your mind.* For a moment, just *freeze-frame ... that picture* (gesturing to a place in front of her) *on the cloud. She's gonna do some dreaming.* Now, *in her dream ... she's gonna suddenly discover herself, surrounded by lots of white fluffy clouds. It's a different cloud.* It's not the same one, *it's a different cloud ...* AND *she's gonna discover that she's a projection. In her dream, she's gonna discover that she's an image that's been projected on to a cloud.* (5 sec.) It's rather strange because *she can look down.* AS *she looks down, she can see a laser down there, that's projecting onto the cloud. She realises that she is an image that is projected by the laser.* It's an interesting dream to have. (7 sec.) So, *in her dream, she ... starts to feel what it feels like to be ... a projection or an image. ... Feels pretty neutral,* doesn't it?

Now it is time for the next step in the process of double dissociation. So far, she has been looking at herself looking at the image of a spider on a cloud. Now she will start looking at the version of herself on the beach who is, in turn, looking up at herself on a cloud. This is a full double dissociation: Brooks suggests this is to happen in a dream, implying that it is a creative and unconscious process. He makes sure she remains dissociated from the image of the spider by telling her that she is on a different cloud and that she can feel neutral there.

Embedded suggestions:

- Now[TA] I want you to[ER] *do some dreaming, do a little bit of dreaming in your mind.*
- For a moment[TA] just[DA] *freeze-frame that picture on the cloud.*
- Now[DM] *in her dream she's gonna suddenly discover herself surrounded by lots of white fluffy clouds.*
- It's rather strange[QA] because *she can look down.*
- So[DM] *in her dream she starts to feel what it feels like to be a projection or an image.*
- *Feels pretty neutral* doesn't it[TQ]?

Direct suggestions:

- *She's gonna do some dreaming.*
- *It's a different cloud.*
- *In her dream, she's gonna discover that she's an image that's been projected on to a cloud.*
- *She realises that she is an image that is projected by the laser.*

Dependent suggestions:

- AS *she looks down - she can see a laser down there.*

Adjunctive suggestions:

- *It's a different cloud -* AND *she's gonna discover that she's a projection.*

Direct statements:

- It's an interesting dream to have.

Vague language:

- Nominalisation: dream, dreaming, projection
- Vague verb: discover
- Loaded word: dream
- Unspecified place: down there
- Unspecified quantity: lots of
- Comparative deletion: it's a different cloud
- No personal pronoun (infinitive): It's an interesting dream to have

Presuppositions:

- Qualifying adjective:
  <u>a little bit</u> of dreaming ⊇ <u>a bit</u> of dreaming ⊇ dreaming

- Qualifying adverb:
  she's gonna <u>suddenly</u> discover herself ⊇ she's gonna discover herself
  it's <u>rather</u> strange ⊇ it's strange
  feels <u>pretty</u> neutral ⊇ feels neutral

- Possessive determiner:
  in <u>her</u> dream ⊇ she has a dream
- Demonstrative determiner:
  <u>that</u> picture ⊇ there is a specific picture
- Change-of-time verb:
  she <u>starts to</u> feel... ⊃ she will continue to feel

Various techniques:

- Enhancing unconscious process: "dreaming"
- Double dissociation: "*she* realises that *she* is an *image that is projected* by the laser"

Client: Mmm.

Brooks: Mmm. ... And she's gonna discover, BECAUSE *she's just a projection and not a real person, she can* **change into anything and become anything** *she wants.* ... So, what is it that she could become? What would you like her to become, to *change from being who she is*? What could she become? Who could she become? Someone else or something else? What would you like to *see her become*? (5 sec.) What comes to mind? *Anybody she'd like to be* ... as a part of this dream?

Client: A baby.

Brooks: A baby. *See her become a baby.* All of the sudden *she feels like a baby, looking out of the cloud. She feels herself as if she is a projected baby, on a cloud, looking down. Strange, interesting experience,* BUT *a very nice feeling, comfortable feeling, very comfortable feeling.*

> So far, Brooks has been predicting and seeding, change and he has built the context to make it happen. Now he actually invites her to change, although still in vague and indirect terms. To her conscious mind, he says "The laser projection can change into anything". To her unconscious, he says "You can change into anything". Note that the suggested change is at the level of identity, not of behaviour. Her response to his question is, perhaps, surprising; she doesn't see herself as a relaxed, confident or strong woman, as Brooks might have expected, but as a baby. Her facial expression and voice tone seem to indicate, however, that this is a positive experience. Why she thinks of a baby is not clear, and Brooks

doesn't ask her. He simply fully accepts her response and utilises it. He keeps her dissociated and suggests positive feelings for the projected baby. Even if she chooses to become a baby now, the seed for a new future identity is planted. Brooks can talk to either of these 'versions' of the client by projecting his voice in different directions and by using different voice tones.

Embedded suggestions:

- <u>All of the sudden</u>[SA] *she feels like a baby looking out of the cloud.*

Questions with an embedded suggestion:

- What would you like her to become, to *change from being who she is*?
- What would you like to *see her become*?

Direct suggestion:

- *See her become a baby.*
- *She feels herself as if she is a projected baby, on a cloud, looking down.*

Adjunctive suggestion:

- *Strange, interesting experience* - BUT *a very nice feeling, comfortable feeling.*

Cause-effect link:

- *And she's gonna discover* - BECAUSE *she's just a projection and not a real person - she can change into anything and become anything she wants.*

Vague language:

- Nominalisation: projection, dream
- Vague verb: discover, change, become
- Loaded word: dream
- Vague adjective: strange, interesting, nice, comfortable
- Unspecified person: a real person, someone else
- Unspecified object/event: something else
- Universal quantifier: anything
- Covering all possibilities: *someone* else or *something* else

Presuppositions:

- Question:
  what could she become? $\supseteq$ she could become something
  who could she become? $\supseteq$ she could become someone
  what comes to mind? $\supseteq$ something comes to mind

- Relative clause:
  what is it that she could become $\supseteq$ she could become something
  to change from being who she is $\supseteq$ she is someone now

- Qualifying adverb:
  she's just a projection $\supseteq$ she's a projection
  very nice comfortable feeling $\supseteq$ nice comfortable feeling

- Demonstrative determiner:
  as a part of this dream $\supseteq$ there is a specific dream

Various techniques:

- Identity change: "who could she become"

Brooks: And now, (making a downward gesture) *let this cloud ... come down, onto the horizon with baby on it, in the dream.* And *in her dream, she experiences the cloud, lowering down onto the beach.* ... And *there on another cloud, is a picture of the spider.* And *the little baby looks across at the spider picture.* And *the spider picture looks back at the baby picture.* And *the spider picture ... looks scaaared. The little spider on the spider picture looks very scared, at the baby*, BECAUSE *the baby is so biiiig*, compared to the little spider. I want you to *watch the little spider start to panic. It can't get out of the cloud. Watch the little spider ... running all over the cloud, it can't get away, it's so scared of the baby.* And *the baby looks over and laughs, thinks it's very funny. ... Watch the baby ... laughing, looking at that little spider running around.* Because little babies, they don't realise. In a way, they have no respect for life, ... little children, you know, they step on the spider without thinking about it, without thinking it's a little life. *The little baby wants to play with it ...* BUT *the little spider is so scared.* How are we gonna *let the little spider go*? How are we gonna, how are we gonna *free the little spider*? Because *the baby wants to play with it.* The baby might hurt it though. *Look at the poor little spider look so scared, so scared of the baby.* (5 sec.)

Brooks has made sure that both the version of herself on the beach and the projected baby can feel comfortable while looking at the spider. He now starts a visualisation process with an interaction between the projected baby and the spider. His words are directed to the adult, dissociated version of herself as if he is telling a story about a baby and the spider. His voice tone, however, is enthusiastic and playful, like he is trying to engage a child in a story. So, he is keeping her 'adult-self' in a state of dissociation with his words while, at the same time, encouraging her 'baby-self' to associate by playing a game with the spider. Within this game, he totally reframes the former situation of her being a child afraid of spiders. Now, the roles are reversed: the spider is afraid of the baby. Her adult dissociated self can easily see that the baby is much bigger than the spider and can understand the logic of the spider being afraid. As her baby self, she can enjoy being called 'biiiiiiig'. Children usually like to be complimented for having grown so big. She can now experience being 'big' compared to the small spider. She now has a different adult (Brooks) as a role model and teacher to the one she had back then (her mother). Brooks playfully puts the baby into the role of threatening perpetrator and the spider into the role of threatened, unfortunate victim. Being the perpetrator implies being powerful. Being the victim implies being harmless. Brooks tells the story playfully and dramatically, appealing to the unconscious childhood desire to participate. He also encourages her dissociated adult self to participate as a resource person, perhaps even as a co-therapist ("How are *we* gonna free the spider?"). Freeing the spider is, of course, a metaphor for freeing herself. This part of the session is a form of metaphorical inner child work, in which the therapist - and the adult self - help the inner child heal and grow.

Embedded suggestions:

- And[DM] now[TA] *let this cloud come down onto the horizon with baby on it, in a dream.*
- And[DM] *in her dream, she experiences the cloud lowering down onto the beach.*
- And[DM] *there on another cloud is a picture of the spider.*
- And[DM] *the little baby looks across at the spider picture.*
- And[DM] *the spider picture looks back at the baby picture.*

- And[DM] *the spider picture looks scared.*
- I want you to[ER] *watch the little spider start to panic.*
- And[DM] *the baby looks over and laughs, thinks it's very funny.*
- Because[DM] *the baby wants to play with it.*

Questions with an embedded suggestion:

- How are we gonna *let the little spider go?*
- How are we gonna *free the spider?*

Direct suggestions:

- *It can't get out of the cloud.*
- *Watch the little spider running all over the cloud, it can't get away, it's so scared of the baby.*
- *Watch the baby laughing, looking at that little spider running around.*
- *Look at the poor little spider look so scared, so scared of the baby.*

Adjunctive suggestions:

- *The little baby wants to play with it* - BUT *the little spider is so scared.*

Cause-effect link:

- *The little spider on the spider picture looks very scared, at the baby* - BECAUSE *the baby is so big.*

Embedded statements:

- Because[DM] little babies they don't realise.
- In a way[SA] they have no respect for life.
- Little children, you know[FV] they step on the spider.
- You know[DM] they step on the spider without thinking about it, without thinking it's a little life.
- The baby might hurt it though[SA].

Vague language:

- Nominalisation: horizon, dream, respect, life
- Vague verb: experiences, panic, realise, play, free, hurt
- Vague adjective: scared, funny, poor

- Loaded word: dream
- Unspecified person: little babies, little children
- Unspecified place: there

Presuppositions:

- Question:
  how are we gonna let the little spider go? ⊇ we are gonna let the little spider go
  how are we gonna free the spider? ⊇ we are gonna free the spider

- Qualifying adverb:
  looks very scared ⊇ looks scared
  the baby is so big ⊇ the baby is big
  it's so scared of the baby ⊇ it's scared of the baby
  thinks it's very funny ⊇ thinks it's funny

- Demonstrative determiner:
  let this cloud come down ⊇ there is a specific cloud

Implications:

- big baby ⊃ powerful baby
- little spider ⊃ harmless spider

Various techniques:

- Reframing: from a 'child being scared of a spider' to 'a spider being scared of a child'
- Metaphor: 'freeing the spider' stands for 'freeing herself'
- Nonverbal implication: being the perpetrator (the client) implies strength; being the victim (the spider) implies weakness

Brooks: Now *you look at the picture of the baby*, BECAUSE *the baby can transform ... back into the woman.* (5 sec.) Now *see her face on the cloud, she looks across at the spider. The spider is even more scared now*. Suddenly *the baby is **all grown up** and big.* (5 sec.) *The little spider is even more scared*, SO MUCH SO ... that *the woman in the cloud ... she starts to feel sorry for the spider, starts to feel sorry for him. It looks so scared.* So ... *she decides*

... *to* ***make it a friend****, to* ***become friends with it****, ... to try and talk to it, make it* ***feel comfortable*****, and not so scared***.* Of course, it can't really hear, BUT she wants to *comfort it and make it* ***feel better****.* Because in her past she knew what it felt like to be scared of something, in her past, something she experienced a lot, in her past, but no more. She doesn't want the little spider to feel scared of her. After all, it's a harmless thing, can't do anything at all, just wants to run away.

> This next scene in the play is also the next step of the therapy; transforming the powerful baby into a powerful woman implies empowering every life phase in between. Furthermore, the play parallels her life history but with the roles reversed. In the past, as she grew up she became more scared. Now, as she grows up, the spider gets more scared. Note the stepwise development of her changing response to spiders: look at it —notice it is scared— feel sorry for it —become friends with it— help it. Her own past fear is now turned into a resource. It helps her sympathise with the spider and understand what she can do to help it. This is a beautiful form of utilisation. Brooks utilises the experience of her past fear to sympathise with and help the spider and, by doing so, help herself. In a way, the problem is utilised to solve the problem. Let's look at the sentence "...something she experienced a lot, in her past, but no more". It is a two-fold suggestion that her problem is over. First, saying she experienced it in the past 'implies' she does not experience it anymore. Then he says the same thing 'explicitly' with the words "but no more". Brooks uses this technique a lot, repeating a suggestion in different ways: implicitly and explicitly; directly and indirectly; literally and metaphorically; and verbally and nonverbally.
>
> Embedded suggestions:
>
> - <u>Now</u>[DM] *see her face on the cloud, she looks across at the spider.*
> - <u>Suddenly</u>[TA] *the baby is all grown up.*
> - <u>So</u>[DM] <u>she decides to</u>[MO] *make it a friend*, to *become friends with it*, to *try and talk to it, make it feel comfortable.*
> - <u>She wants to</u>[MO] *comfort it and make it feel better.*

Adjunctive suggestions:

- Of course, it can't really hear - BUT she wants to *comfort it and make it feel better.*

Cause-effect link:

- Now *you look at the picture of the baby* - BECAUSE *the baby can transform back into the woman.*
- *The little spider is even more scared* - SO MUCH SO that *the woman in the cloud, she starts to feel sorry for the spider.*

Embedded statements:

- <u>Because</u>[DM] in her past she knew what it felt like to be scared of something, in her past, something she experienced a lot, in her past, but no more.
- <u>After all</u>[SA] it's a harmless thing, can't do anything at all, just wants to run away.

Direct suggestions:

- *The spider is even more scared now.*
- *He looks so scared.*

Direct statements:

- She doesn't want the little spider to feel scared of her.

Vague language:

- Vague verb: transform, feel sorry, decide, to become friends, to comfort, experienced
- Vague adjective: harmless, comfortable, scared
- Loaded word: transform
- Unspecified person: the woman
- Unspecified time: in her past
- Unspecified frequency: a lot
- Unspecified object/event: something, (harmless) thing
- Comparative deletion: more scared
- Universal quantifier: anything

Presuppositions:

- Simple presupposition:
  the woman in the cloud ⊇ there is a woman in the cloud

- Repetitive cue word:
  transform back into the woman ⊇ she was a woman before

- Qualifying adverb:
  the spider is even more scared ⊇ the spider is more scared
  all grown up ⊇ grown up
  he looks so scared ⊇ he looks scared
  can't do anything at all ⊇ can't do anything

Implications:

- something she experienced a lot in her past ⊃ she does not experience that anymore
- she starts to feel sorry for the spider ⊃ she will continue to feel sorry for the spider

Various techniques:

- Reframing: the frame of the client's relation with spiders is changed from 'danger and fear' to 'sympathy, friendship, and help'
- Metaphor: 'helping the spider' stands for 'helping herself'

Brooks: So how can she *look after it*? How can she make it ***feel more comfortable and okay***? What sort of things can she say to him? Notice what *thoughts come to mind* now. What *words come to mind that you could say* (5 sec.) *to the little spider*, TO MAKE IT *feel less scared*. What sort of things? What would you have liked to have heard in the past, when you had the problem in the past (gesturing to a place behind her)?

Helping the spider now becomes more specific: it means saying comforting things to the spider. Brooks uses an auditory resource here (words), matching the original, auditory source of the problem (her mother saying, "Run"). He utilises the sensory channel that caused the problem to solve it. Since she doesn't respond readily, Brooks changes his question and asks what she would have liked to have heard in the past. He lets her step out of the spider roleplay for a moment and think about her own needs as a child.

Embedded suggestions:

- *Notice what thoughts come to mind* now[TA].

Questions with an embedded suggestion:

- How can she *look after it*?
- How can she *make it feel more comfortable and okay*?

Cause-effect link:

- What *words come to mind that you could say to the little spider* - TO MAKE IT *feel less scared.*

Vague language:

- Nominalisation: mind, problem
- Vague verb: look after
- Vague adjective: comfortable, okay, scared
- Unspecified time: in the past
- Unspecified object/event: things
- Comparative deletion: less scared
- Permissive: you could

Presuppositions:

- Question:
  how can she look after it? ⊇ she can look after it
  how can she make it feel more...? ⊇ she can make it feel more...
  what sort of things can she say? ⊇ she can say some sort of things
  what would you have liked to have heard? ⊇ you would like to have heard something

- Noun clause:
  notice what thoughts come to mind ⊇ some thoughts come to mind

- Relative clause:

  Words that you could say $\supseteq$ you can say certain words

Implications:

- when you had the problem, in the past $\supset$ you don't have the problem anymore

Client: I'm not going to hurt you.

Brooks: I'm not gonna hurt you. *Say that now to the spider, say it.* ... Because it looks frightened. ... So just *say it in your mind.* And what else would you have liked to have heard in the past, when you had your problem before, in the past (gesturing to a place behind her)? What sort of things would you have liked to have heard then that you could now say to the spider now?

Client: Don't panic.

Brooks: Don't panic. *Say that to the spider*, now.

She can easily answer the questions about what she would have liked to have heard, so Brooks leads her back to the interaction with the spider. He has utilised the little detour to:

- Elicit an auditory resource (Her words: "I'm not going to hurt you.")
- Imply the problem is over (when you had the problem in the past)
- Apply the message for the spider to her inner child

This is another neat example of how the client's response (including no response) can be utilised.

Embedded suggestions:

- So[DM] just[DA] *say it in your mind.*
- *Say that to the spider*, now[TA].

Direct suggestions:

- *Say that now to the spider, say it.*

Embedded statements:

- Because[DM] it looks frightened.

Vague language:

- Nominalisation: problem
- Vague verb: hurt, panic
- Vague adjective: frightened
- Unspecified time: in the past, then
- Unspecified object/event: things
- Permissive: you could

Presuppositions:

- Question:
  what sort of things would you have liked to have heard? ⊇ you would like to have heard some sort of things
- Relative clause:
  things…that you could now say to the spider ⊇ there are things
- Repetitive cue word:
  what else would you have liked to have heard ⊇ there is already something you would have like to have heard

Implications:

- when you had your problem before, in the past ⊃ you don't have your problem anymore

Various techniques:

- Applying resources: "say that now to the spider"

Brooks: Notice *the spider is starting to quieten down* AND somehow *looks friendlier* ... Because you know, you could almost *imagine, it has a little, kind of nice little face.* Well, *like a cartoony face.* You know *like a cartoon.*

Client: Mmm.

Brooks: Also *imagine it having a little face. It looks a little bit shy* at the moment, BUT you can just *look at the corner of its mouth, it's just starting to smile* a little bit. It's not sure whether it can *trust you* or not. And *notice how the two clouds start to get a little bit closer together.* Because somehow *you feel drawn towards that cloud.* ... Don't you want to *help that little thing*? (5 sec.) All it needs is for you, to ***trust it*** ... SO that *it can* ***trust you.*** (8 sec.)

Here Brooks probably sees her accepting and relaxing, and attributes that to the spider in the story. Note that every change in the visualised spider and in any instance of her visualised self is actually a change in her (sitting in the chair) and is noticeable in her minimal cues. Her adult self has given resources to the spider now, in the form of comforting words. Her inner child (the scared part of herself) is receiving those same resources. The effects of that become visible in her minimal cues and Brooks utilises it. He stays within the playful, childlike frame by having her visualise a cartoon-like face on the spider. This makes the spider both human and funny. It is hard to be scared of something with a funny little human face. It is suggested that the spider is shy and unsure about trusting her. This paces and normalises her own possible shyness and insecurity. Clearly, she feels a lot more relaxed and comfortable now, even when she is looking at a spider at close range. However, she might not yet trust these positive feelings. Furthermore, attributing shyness and insecurity to the spider implies, once again, that spiders are harmless. Now, look at the sentence, "All it needs is for you, to trust it so that it can trust you". The explicit link here is "you can trust it — it can trust you". The sentence, however, implies two other important things:

- 'all it needs' implies 'it doesn't need much to help the spider'
- 'all it needs is to trust it' implies 'trusting it is easy'

All of this is not strictly true or logical, but it is made true by suggestion.

Embedded suggestions:

- Because[DM] you know[FV] you could[MO] almost[LS] *imagine it has a little* kind of[LS] *nice little face.*
- Well[DM] *like a cartoony face.*
- You know[DM] *like a cartoon.*
- Also *imagine it having a little face.*

- And[DM] *notice how the two clouds start to get a little bit closer together.*
- Because[DM] *somehow you feel drawn towards that cloud.*

Questions with an embedded suggestion:

- Don't you want to *help that little thing?*

Adjunctive suggestions:

- Notice the spider is starting to *quieten down* - AND somehow *looks friendlier.*
- *It looks a little bit shy* at the moment - BUT you can just *look at the corner of its mouth, it's just starting to smile* a little bit.

Cause-effect link:

- All it needs is for you, to *trust it* - SO that *it can trust you*

Direct statements:

- It's not sure whether it can *trust you* or not.

Vague language:

- Vague verb: quieten (down), imagine, trust, feel drawn
- Vague adjective: cartoony, shy, sure
- Unspecified process: somehow
- Comparative deletion: friendlier, closer
- Permissive: you could, you can

Presuppositions:

- Negative question:
  don't you want to help that little thing ⊇ I think you want to help that little thing
- Noun clause:
  notice how the two clouds start to get a little bit closer ⊇ the two clouds start to get a little bit closer
- Change-of-time verb:
  start to get a little bit closer ⊇ will continue to get close

- Repetitive cues word:
  also imagine $\supseteq$ you already imagined something else
- Qualifying adjective:
  it has a kind of nice little face $\supseteq$ it has a kind of face
- Qualifying adverb:
  somehow looks friendlier $\supseteq$ looks friendlier
  a little bit shy $\supseteq$ shy
  it's just starting to smile $\supseteq$ it's starting to smile
  smile a little bit $\supseteq$ smile
  get a little bit closer $\supseteq$ get closer
- Demonstrative determiner:
  that little thing $\supseteq$ there is a specific little thing
- Pseudo-cleft sentence:
  all it needs is for you to trust it $\supseteq$ it needs something for you

Implications:

- it looks a little bit shy at the moment $\supset$ it will not look shy later

Various techniques:

- Visualisation: "imagine it has a little kind of nice little face"
- Reframing: from 'the client trusting spiders' to 'spiders trusting her'

Brooks: Now ***you have the key*** *to that cloud.* As you can *unlock that cloud* AND *let the spider run away.* But you will discover, WHEN *you unlock it,* it *doesn't want to run away,* BECAUSE it feels it has ***found a friend,*** *someone it can trust, someone who is not going to kill it ... or hurt it.* ... And *someone who is willing ... just to stay there ...* AND *acknowledge it and say:* "***You are my friend***'. You're harmless, I want to *help you* BECAUSE you look so scared. You might even want to *apologise to it.* Sorry *I am human,* sorry ***I am so much bigger than you.*** (13 sec.)

After the stages of helping the spider and becoming his friend, she is now presented with the idea of freeing him. The suggestion 'you have the key to that cloud' is a metaphor for 'you have the key to your prison of fear'. The key is a symbol for opening doors, both literally and figuratively. Letting the spider go is a metaphor for letting her fear go. Brooks takes it one step further. He suggests the spider wants to stay because it has found a friend. The frame of friendship and trust is introduced. Remember the roles are still reversed here and this is actually a metaphor for her trusting spiders. Having her apologise for being so much bigger, puts her in the role of the perpetrator again, implying she has the power.

Embedded suggestions:

- Now[DM] *you have the key to that cloud.*
- But[DM] you will discover[FV] ...it *doesn't want to run away.*
- You might[MO] even want to[MO] *apologise to it.*
- Sorry[TF] *I am human*, sorry[TF] *I am so much bigger.*

Adjunctive suggestions:

- As you can *unlock that cloud* - AND *let the spider run away.*
- Someone who is not going to kill it or hurt it - AND *someone who is willing just to stay there* - AND *acknowledge it and say:* "*You are my friend*".

Dependent suggestion and cause-effect link:

- WHEN *you unlock it - it doesn't want to run away* - BECAUSE *it feels it has found a friend.*

Cause-effect link:

- I want to *help you* - BECAUSE you look so scared.

Direct statement:

- You're harmless.

Vague language:

- Vague verb: unlock, discover, trust, hurt, acknowledge, help, apologise
- Vague adjective: harmless, scared, human
- Unspecified person: a friend, someone

- Permissive: you can, you might

Presuppositions:

- Subordinate clause of time:
  <u>when</u> you unlock it ⊇ you will unlock it

- Qualifying adverb:
  you might <u>even</u> want to apologise ⊇ you might want to apologise

- Demonstrative determiner:
  the key to <u>that</u> cloud ⊇ there is a specific cloud

Implications:

- it has found a friend ⊃ you are its friend

Various techniques:

- Symbolism: 'the key to the cloud' stands for 'the key to her freedom of fear'

Brooks: And maybe even *think of a name for this little spider, some nice friendly little pet name.*

Client: Harry.

Brooks: Harry. ... Harry the spider. Has it got tiny little hairs?

Client: Yeah.

Brooks: Harry, the hairy spider?

Client: Yeah.

Brooks: It could have been *Horace the hairy spider* of course, BUT *Harry the hairy spider. The adventures of Harry the hairy spider.* Hmm. Well, you might *call him by name.* You know what happens when you call people by name, they usually turn around, saying yeah. *Call him, call him by name.* (7 sec.) Some people like to *have little animals as pets*, like a puppy or something, some kind of pet. They like to *call it, and it comes bounding over to you*, you know, *with their tongue hanging out or something.* Children *like that* especially. And you didn't know that ... *all around you*, if you *look hard enough*, you can *find all kinds of wonderful friends, ... little pets.* They will not all be called Harry. Well, they can be if you want. (7 sec.)

Giving the spider a name makes it even more human and makes it even easier for her to feel sympathy and friendship for it. By asking (= suggesting) if the spider has hairs she has to at least imagine that. An animal having hairs suggests it is soft and touchable. Contrasting the spider's name (Harry) with a different name (Horace) and the use of alliteration (Horace, Harry, Hairy) help the client to create a new and positive representation of a spider. The casual remark "The adventures of Harry the hairy spider" is a way of slipping in the word *adventure*, adding another frame for her future encounters with spiders. Brooks further compares the spider to humans and pets, making the idea of it being a friend more and more acceptable. So far, the entire roleplay has been with one spider. Now the frame is extended to many spiders; not directly, but metaphorically, by talking about having a number of friends. And who wouldn't want that? Seeing spiders as friends makes it easier for her to accept the idea of many of them. The statement "They will not all be called Harry" implies they will have other names. This implies they have names in the first place, which again makes them more human. The statement "Well, you can if you want" suggests "they can all be like Harry".

Embedded suggestions:

- And[DM] maybe[SA] even *think of a name for this little spider, some nice friendly little pet name.*
- Well[DM] you might[MO] *call him by name.*
- *It comes bounding over to you,* you know[DM].
- And[DM] you didn't know[FV] that *all around you,* if you *look hard enough,* you can[MO] *find all kinds of wonderful friends, little pets.*

Adjunctive suggestions:

- It could have been *Horace the hairy spider* of course, BUT *Harry the hairy spider.*

Direct suggestions:

- *The adventures of Harry the hairy spider.*
- *Call him, call him by name.*

Embedded statements:

- Well[DM] they can be if you want.
- They like to *call it and it comes bounding over to you*, you know[DM], *with their tongue hanging out or something.*

Direct statements:

- Some people like to *have little animals as pets.*
- Children *like that* especially.

Vague language:

- Nominalisation: adventure
- Vague verb: happen, like
- Vague adjective: nice, friendly
- Unspecified person: people, some people, they
- Unspecified place: all around you
- Unspecified object/event: pets
- Permissive: maybe, you might, you can
- Open-ended: like a puppy or something; some kind of pet

Presuppositions:

- Embedded question:
  you know what happens when you call people by name ⊇ something happens when you call people by name
- Qualifying adjective:
  has it got tiny little hairs ⊇ has it got hairs

Implications:

- they will not all be called Harry ⊃ they have other names ⊃ they have names

Various techniques:

- Analogy: "some people"; "they"
- Association: associating spiders with people and pets

Brooks: Sooo, just *unlock the cloud*, *let Harry just climb out* (gesturing these actions). ... I want you to *watch* ... *watch <name client>, on the beach* now. *She's gonna sit up* AND *talk to Harry*. *You watch her talking to Harry*. Now Harry is not answering, BUT *she can hear him anyway*. So *you listen to Harry answer*. (7 sec.) Now her job is to *make him* ***feel comfortable and not scared***. So just *listen to her saying all those things that she said earlier. Listen to her again, saying those things to him* AND *listen to him answering. He is sooo pleased, so grateful, so pleased*, that at last someone can *listen to him* AND *not hurt him*. (15 sec.) And AS *she sits on the beach, having this conversation with ... Harry, notice how Harry just likes to walk around, walk around her ... in a circle* (drawing an imaginary circle with his right hand). *He's starting to* **feel quite** ... **comfortable** now, with her. *He's not too concerned now, he's not too worried. He is feeling much* **more comfortable**, BECAUSE *he can* **trust** *her*. He knows that she won't suddenly jump and make him scared. She won't suddenly scream and ... frighten him half to death. He knows that she won't suddenly ... stamp on him, or do anything ... dramatic, or anything that might scare or hurt him. He knows that she can ... **treat him** ... **as a friend**. (5 sec.) And you know what friends do? *They* **trust each other**. ... They reeeally **trust each other**. You know, *Harry has lots of* **other friends** as well, AND *they* **trust each other** as well. It won't take long before *word gets out, to all of that community* ... *of fluttery things, or leggy things*, that *all of* **you can be trusted**, *that humans can be trusted* as well. (10 sec.) Now *you watch her now with Harry*. Maybe you can't quite *see his face* at the moment, *see that little smiley, toothy grin he's got, that little smiley, toothy grin.*

It is now time for the next step. She lets the spider out of the cloud and steps out of the cloud herself, although the latter is not suggested explicitly. The double dissociation is brought back to single dissociation. She is kept in her role as the helper of her new friend Harry, who trusts her more and more. Of course, by helping Harry, she is actually helping herself. Now, let's look at the statement, "Now Harry is not answering, but she can hear him anyway. So, you listen to Harry answer." On the surface, this is a contradiction: "Harry is not answering...listen to Harry answer." With multilevel communication, however, it makes sense. To her conscious mind, Brooks is saying, "We know Harry is a spider and he cannot talk"; to the unconscious mind, the message is "Imagine him talking and imagine hearing him". Since the unconscious is not restricted to conscious logic, it can easily imagine this. In this section, the concept of *friendship* is connected to that of *trust,* and both concepts are reinforced with various examples and explanations. The context of her friendship with one spider is enlarged more and more, to include other spiders and other 'fluttery' and 'leggy' things; these creatures are referred to as a community. The word 'community' (a positive nominalisation) implies various things like togetherness, friendship, trust and even love. Brooks does not simply tell her she can be friends with spiders. Given her history, she would probably reject that idea, at least consciously. Instead, he carefully builds a frame of friendship by repeating the same message in various ways: directly and indirectly, explicitly and implicitly, literally and metaphorically. More and more, she is invited, stimulated and even compelled to see spiders as friends. Her conscious mind is engaged in a play and is constantly distracted with complex language patterns. Her unconscious mind receives the same messages over and over again: spiders are harmless; you are powerful; spiders can be friends. Let's look at the sentence, "Maybe you can't quite see his face at the moment". This is a beautiful example of an indirect, implicit and failsafe suggestion. If she is seeing the spider's face, she is doing better than expected so she can be proud. If she is not seeing it, that's okay because this is as suggested. Furthermore "not quite seeing his face at this moment" implies that she will see it properly later. Later, obviously, is a vague description, which could mean a second later. Brooks knows this, so immediately he continues with the suggestion, "see that little smiley, toothy grin." Any resistance or reluctance to seeing the spider's face has been anticipated and normalised before it is suggested. The frame of trust and friendship can be used here because spiders really are harmless. Brooks wouldn't have used this frame for animals that can be dangerous, like dogs.

Embedded suggestions:

- So[DM] just[DA] *unlock the cloud, let Harry just climb out.*
- I want you[ER] to *watch, watch <name client> on the beach* now[DM].
- So[DM] *you listen to Harry answer.*
- Now[DM] her job is to[NP] *make him feel comfortable and not scared.*
- So[DM] just[DA] *listen to her saying all those things that she said earlier.*

- *He is sooo pleased, so grateful, so pleased,* that at last[SA] someone can[MO] *listen to him.*
- *He's starting to feel quite comfortable* now[TA], *with her.*
- *He's not too concerned* now[TA], *he's not too worried.*
- He knows[FV] that she can[MO] *treat him as a friend.*
- It won't take long before[TA] *word gets out to all of that community of fluttery things, or leggy things,* that *all of you can be trusted.*
- Now[DM] *you watch her now with Harry.*
- Maybe[SA] you can't[MO] quite *see his face* at the moment[TA] *see that little smiley, toothy grin he's got.*

Direct suggestions:

- *You watch her talking to Harry.*

Dependent suggestions:

- AS *she sits on the beach... - notice how Harry just likes to walk around.*

Adjunctive suggestions:

- *She's gonna sit up* - AND *talk to Harry.*
- Now Harry is not answering - BUT *she can hear him anyway.*
- *Listen to her again, saying those things to him* - AND *listen to him answering.*
- Someone can *listen to him* - AND *not hurt him.*
- *Harry has lots of other friends* as well - AND *they trust each other* as well.

Cause-effect links:

- He is *feeling much more comfortable* - BECAUSE *he can trust her.*

Direct statements:

- He knows that she won't suddenly jump and make him scared.
- She won't suddenly scream and frighten him half to death.
- He knows that she won't suddenly stamp on him, or do anything dramatic, or anything that might scare or hurt him.
- They *trust each other.*

Vague language:

- Nominalisation: job, conversation, community
- Vague verb: hurt, trust, frighten, scare, treat, gets (out)
- Loaded word: community
- Ambiguous verb: unlock
- Vague adjective: comfortable, scared, pleased, grateful
- Unspecified person: someone, he, friends, they
- Unspecified time: it won't take long
- Unspecified object/event: those things, anything dramatic, the word, fluttery things, leggy things
- Comparative deletion: much more comfortable
- Universal quantifier: all of that community; all of you
- Permissive: maybe

Presuppositions:

- Noun clause:
  you know what friends do ⊇ friends do something

- Relative clause:
  that toothy grin (that) he's got ⊇ he's got that toothy grin

- Repetitive cues word:
  listen to her again ⊇ you listened to her before

- Qualifying adverb:
  Harry just likes to walk around ⊇ Harry likes to walk around
  feel quite comfortable ⊇ feel comfortable
  he's not too concerned ⊇ he's not concerned
  he's not too worried ⊇ he's not worried
  she won't suddenly jump ⊇ she won't jump
  they really trust each other ⊇ they trust each other

- Possessive determiner:
  now her job is to ⊇ she has a job

Implications:

- you can't quite see his face <u>at the moment</u> ⊃ you might/will be able to see his face later

Various techniques:

- Dissociation: "I want you to *watch <name client>*"

Client: Mmm.

Brooks: So just *watch her put out her hand.* He's only a little thing, so he's gonna have a bit of effort trying to crawl on to her hand. Just *watch her do that now.* And *watch him crawl onto her hand*, like ***close friends***. You know, when ***you're with a close friend****, you walk along hand-in-hand.*

Client: Mmm.

Brooks: Here you are, *hand in leg.* ... Just *watch him crawl onto her hand.* And *she's gonna lift it up a little bit*, AND *look into his little furry eyes* (puts on a childlike voice). Poor little thing, little toothy embarrassed grin. He looks almost embarrassed to be there. He says, "How could I make such a fool of myself?" That's what he's saying AS *he looks up to you.* "How could I make such a fool of myself? *You're lovely. You're not going to hurt me.*" He feels a bit embarrassed I think. You know that expression, AS *you look at his face.*

Client: Mmm.

Brooks: Hmm. He says: "Please don't leave me. Look after me somewhere. Find somewhere for me … to live. In your garden or somewhere like that please, *take me home.* Look after me. If you do, I'll tell all my friends, ... that *you can be trusted.*" (5 sec.) So, what do you want to tell him? Do you want to *look after him*?

Client: Yeah.

Brooks: Okay. *Tell him that* now *in your mind.* (9 sec.)

> Now comes the next step in the steadily growing friendship between Harry the spider and the client. Still dissociated, she sees herself put out her hand, allowing the spider to crawl onto it. The frame of friendship is further enriched: they are now *close* friends. Brooks then suggests the spider is embarrassed about making a fool of himself. This is a way of

pacing or anticipating her possible embarrassment about making a fool of herself for a long time. It is also another way of making the spider even more harmless. The play continues, and Harry now asks her for help and a place to live. This matches her cry for help and her desire for a safe home as expressed at the beginning of the session. The *me* in the embedded suggestion "*Take me home*" refers to Harry the spider in the context of the play. Her unconscious mind, however, may interpret Brooks' suggestion *take me home* almost literally, as in: take *me, Stephen Brooks,* home; *take my voice, my image, my touch or any other aspect of me.* Suggesting that the client take something of the therapist home is an Ericksonian way of reinforcing therapeutic effects after the session[53]. By now, the client's relationship with spiders has been totally reframed. It began as a strong negative relationship based on fear, with the spider as the imagined perpetrator and her as the victim. By now, the relationship is one of friendship, trust and care. The spider is now the small, foolish and helpless victim and the client has become the big, powerful and loving caretaker.

Embedded suggestions:

- So[DM] just[DA] *watch her put out her hand.*
- Just[DA] *watch her do that* now[TA].
- And[DM] *watch him crawl onto her hand, like close friends.*
- Just[DA] *watch him crawl onto her hand.*
- *Tell him that* now[TA] *in your mind.*

Dependent suggestions:

- WHEN *you're with a close friend - you walk along hand-in-hand.*
- That's what he's saying - AS *he looks up to you.*
- You know that expression - AS *you look at his face.*

Adjunctive suggestions:

- *She's gonna lift it up a little bit* - AND *look into his little furry eyes.*

[53] Milton Erickson often said to his clients: "my voice will go with you".

Embedded statement:

- He feels a bit embarrassed I think[TF].
- That's what he's saying[Q] … "*You're lovely. You're not going to hurt me.*"
- He says[Q]: "..*take me home*.. you can be trusted."

Direct statements:

- He's only a little thing, so he's gonna have a bit of effort trying to crawl on to her hand.
- He looks almost embarrassed to be there.

Vague language:

- Nominalisation: effort, expression
- Vague verb: hurt, look after, trusted
- Vague adjective: poor, embarrassed, lovely
- Loaded word: fool
- Unspecified person: close friends, a close friend
- Unspecified place: somewhere
- Unspecified object/event: that
- Open-ended: in your garden or something like that
- Mind reading: he feels a bit embarrassed I think

Presuppositions:

- Question:
  what do you want to tell him? $\supseteq$ you want to tell him something

- Qualifying adjective:
  close friends $\supseteq$ friends

- Change-of-place verb:
  please don't leave me $\supseteq$ you are with me

- Reverse pseudo-cleft sentence:
  that's what he's saying $\supseteq$ he's saying something

Implications:

- do you want to look after him? ⊃ he needs to be looked after

Various techniques:

- Dissociation: "*watch her* put out her hand"
- Symbol: 'walking hand in hand' stands for 'friendship'
- Metaphor: 'spider's embarrassment' stands for 'client's possible embarrassment'

Brooks: Now, *put him down again.* And *watch him run around, he's so excited.* Look! His little legs can't keep up with him. He's *sooo excited* running everywhere, look! Leaping up and down, kicking his little legs. Leaping over little pebbles. *Look, he is going crazy. Put your hand down, he'll leap over your hand. You watch … like a leapfrog over your hand. There he goes. And back the other way, here it comes again* (Brooks whistles). *Over the top again. And here he comes another way, up over the top. Over and over your fingers, look. Here now, in and out, over and back onto the ground again, onto the sand. And he comes, here he comes again, climbing over your fingers* (gesturing the movement with his hand), *back down the other side.* He's so excited. Have you ever seen such an excited spider before? So happy … so happy … to have that friend, mmm. (10 sec.)

This is another step in the relationship between the client and Harry the spider. After building friendship, trust and care, it is time for joy and happiness. She is still watching herself playing with the spider. This part of the play appeals to her childhood memories of play, joy and happiness: an important resource for overcoming her fear. After using her adult resources of trust, friendship and care, her childhood resources of playfulness, excitement and craziness are elicited. Letting the spider go crazy also refers to the beginning of the session where she talked about herself going crazy on seeing spiders. Craziness is reframed as something positive now. Referring to something that came up at the beginning enhances amnesia about the session.

Embedded suggestions:

- <u>Now</u>[TA] *put him down again.*

- <u>And</u>[DM] *watch him run around, he's so excited.*

Direct suggestions:

- *Look! His little legs can't keep up with him…*
- *Put your hand down, he'll leap over your hand.*
- *You watch, like a leapfrog over your hand.*
- *There he goes. And back the other way…*

Direct statements:

- He's so excited.
- So happy, so happy to have that friend.

Vague language:

- Nominalisation: way
- Vague adjective: excited, crazy
- Loaded word: crazy
- Unspecified person: that friend
- Unspecified place: up and down, in and out, another way, over the top
- Universal quantifier: everywhere
- No personal pronoun: so happy

Presuppositions:

- Repetitive cue word:
  here it comes <u>again</u> ⊇ it came before

- Qualifying adverb:
  he's <u>so</u> excited ⊇ he's excited
  <u>so</u> happy ⊇ happy

- Demonstrative determiner:
  <u>that</u> friend ⊇ there is a specific friend

Various techniques:

- Metaphor: 'excited and happy spider' stands for 'excited and happy client'

Brooks: Now ... here … I'd like you to *start to ... move towards your own body* again ... (gesturing with his right hand). You probably have already. *Climb into your body, to <name client>'s body*, SO *you're sitting there* AND start to *feel how good it feels ... to be her. Feel, how good it feels to be her.* You saw her do all of that. You saw her with that spider. ... You saw her, how good she felt AND I want you to *feel those good feelings* as well. *You step into her body* AND *really feel all of those good feelings. Put down your hand* AND *let him do some more leapfrogging. Here it comes, little legs going right crazy. Over it goes, hmmm, back on the other side like a little obstacle course.* (Brooks looks at her fingers) Next time you should *wear nail polish*, you can *use it like a slide.* You know, *from the back of the fingers, down the slide*, weeeeehh. Perhaps *that's fun.* (15 sec.)

The next step of the process is ending the dissociation. Brooks lets her return to her body again. Whether that is on the beach or in the chair is left open. Because she hardly speaks, and her body is very still, he is not sure where she is in terms of dissociation-association. To avoid a mismatch, he mentions the possibility she already is in her body. All the good feelings that she observed (dissociation) in herself on the beach can now be felt in her own body (association). Brooks also lets her experience the game of leapfrogging in the associated state. Let's look at the suggestion, "Next time you should wear nail polish". This implies there will be a next time, i.e. that she will play this game again[54]. Nail polish also has associations of fun, beauty, and control (she is the one putting it on). This is in contrast to her old associations of being out of control when seeing an 'ugly' spider.

Embedded suggestions:

- Now[TA] here[PA] I'd like you[ER] to *start to move towards your own body.*
- I want you to[ER] *feel those good feelings* as well.
- Really[SA] *feel all of those good feelings.*
- Next time[TA] you should[MO] *wear nail polish.*
- You can[MO] *use it like a slide.*
- You know[DM] *from the back of the fingers, down the slide.*

[54] Just in case she still experiences fear or in case it comes back in the future.

- Perhaps[SA] *that's fun.*

Direct suggestions:

- *Feel, how good it feels to be her.*
- *Here it comes, little legs going right crazy…*

Adjunctive suggestions:

- You saw her, how good she felt - AND I want you to *feel those good feelings* as well.
- *You step into her body* - AND *really feel all of those good feelings.*
- *Put down your hand* - AND *let him do some more leapfrogging.*

Direct statements:

- You probably have already.
- You saw her do all of that.
- You saw her with that spider.

Cause-effect link and adjunctive suggestion:

- *Climb into your body, to <name client>'s body* - SO *you're sitting there* - AND *start to feel how good it feels to be her.*

Vague language:

- Nominalisation: fun
- Loaded word: crazy
- Unspecified place: here, on the other side
- Unspecified object/event: all of that
- Ambiguity (homonym): right crazy
- Mind reading: you probably have already
- Permissive: perhaps

Presuppositions:

- Noun clause:
  feel how good it feels to be here $\supseteq$ it feels good to be here

- Change-of-time verb:
  start to move towards your own body again ⊇ you can continue to move towards your own body

- Repetitive cue word:
  start to move towards your own body again ⊇ you were near or in your own body before
  I want you to feel those good feelings as well ⊇ someone else already has those good feelings

- Ordinal numeral:
  next time you should wear nail polish ⊇ there will be a next time

- Demonstrative determiner:
  that spider ⊇ there is a specific spider

Various techniques:

- Association: "climb into your body"

Brooks: Well it's now time to *say goodbye to Harry* for a while. What you should do, is *look at him and tell him ... that you'll find him again. You'll look out for him. You'll go looking for him, and his brothers and his friends ... and his sisters.* He has a whole family, you know, somewhere. And families are important. It's always important to have a good family, to have a mother, to have a mother you can trust ... and love. It's so important. And he is just the same, he's got a mother somewhere. ... A family is so important. And *you'll find all of his friends.* Some of them will be very pleased to see you. You know, word spreads reeeally very quickly ... in the insect world. It gets around so quick. And they will be so pleased to see you. So, *you've got some hunting to do, some good friendship hunting.* Go out AND *find there some good friends. You'll find them* if you *look hard enough.* (10 sec.)

The session gradually comes towards closure here. The frame of friendship and community is extended even more: to family and to brothers and sisters. Harry is indirectly defined as a representative of spiders in general, transferring the frame of friendship to the outside world. Introducing the mother creates another similarity between the client and the spider: both have a mother. Again, this refers back to the beginning of the session where the client talked about her mother, so it enhances amnesia. The context of spiders is once more enlarged, this time to encompass the insect world. Now, let's look at that statement "word spreads really very quickly in the insect world". To her conscious mind, this is funny, and it makes sense in the created spider fantasy. To her unconscious, it can mean different things. Note that Brooks pauses after the word 'quickly'. During the pause, her conscious mind will interpret "the word spreads quickly" in the context of the play, or wait for further information. Her unconscious, however, will take it as a suggestion to 'spread word quickly'. Out of context, this is a vague suggestion. In the larger context of her being in therapy with Brooks to overcome her fear, she could unconsciously interpret it as a suggestion to 'spread his word'(i.e. any of the positive nominalisations he has given her) into her future and into the various contexts of her life. As such, her unconscious has started to follow this suggestion of 'spreading the word' in the way it understands it, and it will continue to do so when Brooks finishes the sentence with "in the insect world". All of this happens in a couple of seconds and is just one example of the process of indirect, vague and multilevel communication that Brooks demonstrates in this session. The task of hunting puts her in the role of perpetrator once more. The phrase 'friendship hunting' not only tells her what to hunt but also how to interpret hunting (as a friendly act).

Embedded suggestions:

- Well[DM] it's now time[TA] to *say goodbye to Harry* for a while[TA].
- What you should do[MO], is *look at him and tell him that you'll find him again.*
- And[DM] *you'll find all of his friends.*
- So[DM] *you've got some hunting to do, some good friendship hunting.*

Direct (posthypnotic) suggestions:

- *You'll look out for him.*
- *You'll go looking for him, and his brothers and his friends and his sisters.*
- *You'll find them,* if you *look hard enough.*

Adjunctive suggestions:

- Go out - AND *find there some good friends.*

Embedded statements:

- He has a whole family, you know[DM] somewhere[PA].
- And[DM] families are important.
- It's always important[QA] to have a good family, to have a mother you can trust and love.
- And[DM] he is just the same, he's got a mother somewhere.
- You know[DM] word spreads really very quickly in the insect world.
- And[DM] they will be so pleased to see you.

Direct statement:

- It's so important.
- A family is so important.
- Some of them will be very pleased to see you.
- It gets around so quick.

Vague language:

- Nominalisation: friendship, hunting
- Vague verb: trust, love, hunt
- Vague adjective: important, good, pleased, quick
- Vague adverb: quickly
- Unspecified person: brothers, sisters, friends, whole family, a mother, some of them
- Lost performative: families are important
- Comparative deletion: the same
- Unspecified place: somewhere, out, there
- Universal quantifier: always

Presuppositions:

- Pseudo-cleft sentence:

what you should do is look at him $\supseteq$ you should do something

- Qualifying adverb:
  word spreads really very quickly $\supseteq$ word spreads very quickly $\supseteq$ word spreads quickly $\supseteq$ word spreads
  it gets around so quick $\supseteq$ it gets around quick $\supseteq$ it gets around

Brooks: Just *spend some time* now, *thinking about, what you've achieved* here. *Notice how you felt. Notice how you used to feel before* if you'd have thought of a spider. *Notice how you feel now.* Just to *spend some time thinking about that.* And WHILE *you are doing that now*, <name client>, I'm going to talk, BUT *you don't have to listen to my voice or what I say* (gesturing towards her). Just *spend time thinking about what you've been doing.*

Brooks gives her the task of thinking about what she has been doing and what she has achieved during the session. The implication is that 'she' has done the work and that she has succeeded. The sentences "Notice how you felt. Notice how you feel now", not only suggest she 'notice' the difference (consciously) but also to 'reinforce' that difference (unconsciously). He talks to the audience now for a couple of minutes, making some suggestions to the client about looking for friends, the effectiveness of the session and her use of it for her daughter.

Embedded suggestions:

- Just[DA] *spend some time* now[DM] *thinking about what you've achieved* here[PA].
- Just[DA] to *spend some time thinking about that.*
- Just[DA] *spend time thinking about what you've been doing.*

Direct suggestions:

- *Notice how you felt.*
- *Notice how you used to feel before.*
- *Notice how you feel now.*

Dependent/adjunctive suggestion:

- WHILE *you are doing that now*, <name client> - I'm going to talk - BUT *you don't have to listen to my voice.*

Vague language:

- Vague verb: to achieve
- Unspecified time: some time, time
- Unspecified object/event: that

Presuppositions:

- Noun clause:
  thinking about what you've achieved here ⊇ you have achieved something
  thinking about what you've been doing ⊇ you have been doing something
- Subordinate clause of time:
  whilst you are doing that ⊇ you are doing that – or will be doing that

Implications:

- notice how you used to feel before ⊃ you don't feel this way anymore

Various techniques:

- Talking to others: talking to the audience

Brooks: Now in a few moments tiiime ... I'm gonna lift your right arm into the air. WHEN I lift it into the air ... you'll notice *it starts to become a little ... rigid ... and fixed in the air.* And you can *be curious about that*, AS *it happens.* On the count of three, when I reach the number three ... I'll lift that arm into the air. And AS it happens, *notice the feeling in it.* Here we go (takes her right arm at the wrist), one, two, three (he supports the arm at the elbow with his other hand but lets go of the wrist and, leaving the arm up in the air, he pushes it gently in various directions to enhance catalepsy) that's it, that's it. *Those fingers are going to straighten out, straighten out, straighten out. They will become rigid.* Almost *as if there is an iron bar inserted in it* now, *as if it there is an iron bar inserted in your arm*, that's it, *rigid, rigid.* Almost as if it could snap so quickly if you tried to bend it. *It's sooo stiff and rigid, sooo strong.* You know, you maybe have heard those stories of mothers *suddenly having incredible strength* when they need to, in emergency situations. They can *have access to incredible strength. That arm has got all of that strength in it* now. *It's so strong*, it could *become so rigid.* THE HARDER *you try to bend it*, THE MORE ... *rigid it becomes.* THE HARDER *you try and bend it*, THE MORE *rigid it becomes.* It's almost as if it could snap. In a moment, I'm gonna count to three, WHEN I reach the number three, THE HARDER *you try to bend that arm*, THE MORE *rigid it becomes. So rigid, so rigid* almost *as if there's an iron bar, running along that arm, that's just sooo rigid, soo rigid, so rigid.* On the count to three, WHEN I reach the number three, *you can try and bend that arm* AND THE HARDER *you try to bend that arm*, THE MORE *rigid it becomes* ... THE MORE *rigid it becomes.* One, *getting ready to try*, two, *getting ready to try. Becoming more rigid* even now AS I talk, three *becoming so rigid, so rigid, so rigid, like an iron bar.* THE HARDER *you try and bend it*, THE MORE *rigid it becomes.* That's it, that's it, THE HARDER *you try*, *the more rigid*, THE MORE *stiff.* THE HARDER *you try*, that's it, THE *STIFFER it becomes*, THE HARDER *you try.* You can *really try harder and harder* AND *it becomes more and more rigid.* That's it. THE MORE *effort you put in*, THE *HARDER it becomes*, THE *HARDER it becomes.* That's it, *really try hard. Really try hard, it becomes so rigid.* That's it, *so rigid*, THE HARDER *you try* THE MORE *rigid it becomes. So rigid ... so rigid.* And this is something that may surprise you. It may surprise you BECAUSE in the past (pointing behind her), this didn't happen, BUT now (pointing in front of her), *see what you can do ... See what you can do, see what I can dooo, I can do with your mind* AND you will *no longer have your old fear.* It is gone, it's a thing of the past, it no longer exists. Now you can *feel comfortable and confident and happy with any insects as spiders, moths, any long-legged.* You can *feel quite comfortable and relaxed and comfortable with it. No fear at all, all in the past, you'll feel verrry verrry comfortable and relaxed.* This arm IS A DEMONSTRATION OF what I can do with your mind using hypnosis. And then *it relaxes* AS I grab it (takes her arm at the wrist from above and guides it down to her lap). *Your arm just relaxes* AND *goes floppy* now (lets go of her arm and touches her on the shoulder). (Lowers his voice and starts to talk more slowly). *Deeper, deeper relaxed, all the way down.* You're doing verrry, verrry well <name client>, verrry, very well. Well done, very well, *deeper relaxed, aand deeper, aand deeper relaxed aand deeper.* That's it, doing very, very well (lets go of her shoulder and turns to the audience).

Now Brooks comes back to the beginning of the session in a different way. Before, when he mentioned the spider going crazy and having a mother, he did so verbally. Now he does it verbally and nonverbally by creating arm catalepsy again. Here, at the end of the session, rapport is stronger, and she's in a deeper trance. This means he can be more direct and even authoritarian. The latter also matches her thinking style: external reference. Brooks uses repetition (rigid – rigid), metaphor (iron bar), the law of reversed effort (the harder you try, the more rigid it becomes) and complimenting ('doing very well'). He first induces the arm catalepsy and then utilises it as proof: proof of his power and the power of hypnosis. So, the conscious mind can believe that he or hypnosis solved the problem, utilising her external locus of control. Meanwhile, her unconscious can realise more and more that she did it. It has been supported in believing this throughout the session with countless ratifications, compliments and repeated gratitude.

Embedded suggestions:

- You'll notice[FV] *it starts to become a little rigid and fixed in the air.*
- Almost[LS] *as if there is an iron bar inserted in it* now[TA].
- You know[DM], you maybe[SA] have heard those stories of mothers *suddenly having incredible strength.*
- They can[MO] *have access to incredible strength.*
- *That arm has got all of that strength in it* now[TA].
- *It's so strong,* it could[MO] *become so rigid.*
- *So rigid, so rigid* almost[LS] *as if there's an iron bar, running along that arm, that's just so rigid, so rigid, so rigid.*
- You can[MO] *try and bend that arm.*
- Almost[LS] *as if there's an iron bar, running along* that *arm.*
- One[A] *getting ready to try,* two[A] *getting ready to try…* three[A] *becoming so rigid.*
- You can[MO] *really try harder.*
- Now[TA] you can[MO] *feel comfortable and confident and happy with any insects as spiders, moths, any long legged.*
- You can[MO] *feel quite comfortable and relaxed and comfortable with it.*
- And[DM] then *it relaxes* as I grab it.

Direct suggestions:

- *Those fingers are going to straighten out.*
- *They will become rigid.*
- *It's so stiff and rigid, so strong.*
- *So rigid, so rigid.*
- *Really try hard, it becomes so rigid.*
- *One, getting ready to try, two, getting ready to try, becoming more rigid… three becoming so rigid, so rigid, so rigid, like an iron bar.*
- *No fear at all, all in the past, you'll feel very very comfortable and relaxed.*
- *Deeper, deeper relaxed, all the way down.*

Dependent suggestions:

- WHEN I lift it into the air - you'll notice *it starts to become a little rigid.*
- You can *be curious about that* - AS *it happens.*
- AS it happens - *notice the feeling in it.*
- *Becoming more rigi*d even now - AS I talk.
- And then *it relaxes* - AS I grab it.

Adjunctive suggestions:

- You can *really try harder and harder* - AND *it becomes more and more rigid.*
- In the past, this didn't happen - BUT now *see what you can do.*
- *See what you can do, see what I can do, I can do with your mind* - AND *you will no longer have your old fear.*
- *Your arm just relaxes* - AND *goes floppy* now.

Adjunctive suggestions and cause-effect link:

- It may surprise you - BECAUSE in the past this didn't happen - BUT now *see what you can do.*

Explanatory link:

- This arm - IS A DEMONSTRATION OF what I can do with your mind using hypnosis.

Law of reversed effort:

- THE HARDER *you try to bend it* - THE MORE *rigid it becomes.*
- THE HARDER *you try* - THE MORE *rigid* - THE MORE *stiff.*
- THE HARDER *you try*, that's it - THE STIFFER it becomes - THE HARDER *you try.*
- THE MORE *effort you put in* - THE *HARDER it becomes.*

Dependent suggestions and law of reversed effort:

- WHEN I reach the number three - THE HARDER *you try to bend that arm* - THE MORE *rigid it becomes.*

Embedded statements:

- <u>Almost</u>[LS] as if it could snap so quickly if you tried to bend it.
- <u>It's almost</u>[LS] as if it could snap.
- <u>And</u>[DM] this is something that may surprise you.

Direct statements:

- It is gone, it's a thing of the past, it no longer exists.

Vague language:

- Nominalisation: story, emergency, access, strength, fear, demonstration, mind, hypnosis
- Vague verb: surprise, relaxes
- Vague adjective: curious, incredible, strong, old, comfortable, confident, happy, relaxed
- Vague adverb: quickly
- Loaded word: incredible, hypnosis
- Unspecified person: mothers, they
- Unspecified time: in a few moments time, the past
- Unspecified object/event: that, this, something
- Comparative deletion: deeper, harder
- Unspecified place: in the air
- No personal pronoun (dummy subject): there is an iron bar inserted in it now

- No personal pronoun (gerund): getting ready to try…becoming more rigid
- Ambiguity (of scope): very comfortable and relaxed
- Permissive: you can, maybe

Presuppositions:

- Subordinate clause of time:
  you can be curious about that as it happens ⊇ it will happen
  when I lift it into the air ⊇ I will lift it into the air

- Factive verb:
  notice the feeling in it ⊇ there will be a feeling in it

- Demonstrative determiner:
  those stories of mothers ⊇ there are specific stories
  that strength ⊇ there is a specific strength

- Qualifying adjective:
  having incredible strength ⊇ having strength

- Relative clause:
  this is something that may surprise you ⊇ something may surprise you

- Noun clause:
  see what you can do ⊇ you can do something
  see what I can do ⊇ I can do something

- Qualifying adverb:
  so rigid ⊇ rigid
  feel quite comfortable ⊇ feel comfortable
  your arm just relaxes ⊇ your arm relaxes
  very comfortable and relaxed ⊇ comfortable and relaxed

Implications:

- try to bend that arm ⊃ you can't bend that arm

Various techniques:

- Symbol: 'iron bar' stands for 'rigidity'
- Ratifying nonverbal response: "that's it"
- Dissociation: "*those* fingers"; "*that* arm"
- Complimenting: "well done"; "doing very, very well"

Brooks now turns to the group and explains his use of direct suggestion in this part of the session. He also mentions it is important to capitalise on belief systems. He means the beliefs of the client here, but he doesn't specify which beliefs because she can hear him, and he doesn't want her to start thinking about her beliefs at this time. If, for example, she becomes (too) aware of her external reference (believing that other people know better), she might begin to doubt Brooks' expertise and power; she might also question the steps taken, including their effects. Obviously, that is to be avoided.

Brooks: (touches her on the shoulder) Just *go deeper relaxed, deeeeper relaxed.* You're doing very, very well. You know, you've been through all of those steps now. There's one more step to go. And that step is down to you. That step is for you to *step out ... of this room ... in a few minutes time* AND *find yourself one of those friends.* And this is the next step AND that's the final step for you. For you to *step out of the door,* AND *find yourself one of these friends* AND *to let me know, or someone else know, here, how ... great that felt.*

Here Brooks helps her bring her inner changes to the external world and to her real life. First, he reminds her of the steps she has already taken. Then he defines her behaviour in the external world as only one step, the final step of a sequence. This way, the step seems much smaller and easier for her. Remember: a change in behaviour is only as big or difficult as it is perceived to be. The session is almost finished now, but still, Brooks' sentences are loaded with suggestion and implication utilising therapy time to its fullest. Just look at the last sentences of this piece: *...step out of the door, and find yourself one of these friends, and to let me know, or someone else know, here, how great that felt.* It starts with a simple behavioural instruction (step out of the door), which is linked to a therapeutic suggestion (find yourself one of these friends), which is, in turn, connected to pseudo orientation in time (let me know how great it felt).

The option of letting someone else know is a way of making the suggestion valid in case she cannot —or doesn't want to— let Brooks know. The word 'here' is ambiguous, a homophone for 'here' (in this place) or 'hear' (what I say). The indirect suggestion "how great that felt" implies it will feel great. The idea of letting Brooks know how it went is also a way for her to stay in touch with him —at least in her mind— while performing the task of finding spiders.

Embedded suggestions:

- Just[DA] *go deeper relaxed, deeper relaxed.*

Adjunctive suggestions:

- That step is for you to *step out of this room in a few minutes time* - AND *find yourself one of those friends.*
- This is the next step - AND that's the final step for you.
- For you to *step out of the door* - AND *find yourself one* of these *friends* - AND *to let me know...how great that felt.*

Embedded statements:

- You know[FV], you've been through all of those steps now[DM].
- And[DM] that step is down to you.

Direct statements:

- There's one more step to go.

Vague language:

- Nominalisation: step
- Vague adjective: deep, great
- Unspecified time: in a few minutes time
- Unspecified person: one of those friends, someone else
- Comparative deletion: deeper
- No personal pronoun (dummy subject): *there's* one more step to go.
- Ambiguity (homophone): here/hear

Presuppositions:

- Demonstrative determiner:
  <u>that</u> step is down to you ⊇ there is a specific step
  one of <u>those</u> friends ⊇ there are specific friends

- Ordinal numeral:
  the <u>next</u>/<u>final</u> step ⊇ you have already taken steps

- Noun clause:
  Let me know…<u>how great that felt</u> ⊇ that will feel great

Various techniques:

- Complimenting: you're doing very, very well

Brooks: I would like you now, to *look into the eyes of your child.* ... 19 months?

Client: Yeah.

Brooks: *Look into those eyes.* Those eyes are telling you something. Don't they always tell you something those eyes, beautiful eyes. *Look into those eyes* now. Because what you've just done for yourself, now, you've also done for that child, that child's future. Now your mom couldn't help it back then, when she had her problem. You couldn't help learning it. That was just something that happened BUT that child is never having ... never gonna have to learn what you've been through in the past. And that is the gift that you can give your child. Something very special. *Look into those eyes* now, AND *give that gift to your child.* That is something so special. And know that child will never know about it, never realise what you gave it back here. I was thinking that the best gifts are the ones, that you don't actually get appreciation for, the ones you give anonymously almost (smiling, turning to the audience). You don't do it out of selfishness, or wanting kind of, you know, some kind of thanks. You just give it. It's lovely to be able to do that for your own child. Of course, you give many gifts to your child, right? Just being you, just being her mother. That's such a gift. (15 sec.)

> Brooks does many things in this section. Let's look at "Those eyes are telling you something. Don't they always tell you something those eyes." He creates a posthypnotic suggestion here. Having a nineteen-month-old baby, she will obviously look into her child's eyes countless times in

the upcoming years. Since the original problem had a systemic nature involving her mother and her daughter, this is a perfect posthypnotic trigger for her new response. First, he gives her the trigger (those eyes), leaving the response open (are telling you *something*). Then he turns it into a posthypnotic suggestion. The rhetorical question "Don't they always tell you something" presupposes "I think they always tell you something". Then he gives her the posthypnotic response (what you have done for yourself...give that gift to your child). So, every time she looks into her daughter's eyes, she will unconsciously be reminded of what she achieved in the session: feeling comfortable in the presence of spiders or other insects; a general state of comfort, relaxation, confidence and fun; and ideas of trust, friendship and love. This is a nice example of the indirect way Brooks works. A direct posthypnotic suggestion would have been something like "Every time you look into your daughter's eyes you will realise that spiders are friends". Although this could work, it might also cause her to think about it consciously and perhaps question it. So, Brooks delivers the posthypnotic suggestion indirectly, hidden in a visualisation about her daughter. This present to her daughter has multiple functions. Overtly it is a gift for her daughter, and the fact that her daughter will not develop the same fear is probably one of the greatest benefits of this session. Covertly, it creates a systemic change of roles. In the problem frame, the client was the child whose mother taught her to be afraid of spiders. In the solution frame, she is the mother who teaches her own daughter to be friends with spiders. Having the role of teacher implies that she has learned something herself. Furthermore, teaching this reinforces her own learning and brings it into the future. Anyone who has been in the role of teacher, trainer or tutor knows that teaching increases your own knowledge and skills about the topic that you teach. So, is there anything else we can say about this section? Yes, there is! Just look at the sentence, "It's lovely to be able to *do that for your own child*." To whom is Brooks referring here? Why doesn't he say, "your daughter"? Well, to her conscious mind he is referring to her daughter. To her unconscious mind, however, it may mean her daughter or her own inner child. Although the session is almost finished, the inner work might go on for a while. She might need to continue helping her inner child and this suggestion encourages her to do that. Another thing Brooks does here is to normalise what happened in the past and defuse any blame. He does this by suggesting her mother couldn't help it and that she couldn't help it. As far as the her daughter is concerned, he suggests that she has already given her many other gifts, just by being her mother. He makes it clear that there is no need for her to feel guilty about any aspect of her (past) problem.

Brooks has taken a strong leading role in this session, utilising the client's thinking style: external reference and external locus of control. He has guided her through a visualisation and hypnotic desensitisation in which she was relatively passive. He chose the images for her to visualise, outlined the steps for her to take and talked her through the process. As usual, he closely monitored her responses and adapted his communication wherever needed. Now, near the end of the session, he starts to subtly diminish his role by talking about anonymous gifts, gifts you don't need to be thanked for. Overtly, he is talking about her gifts to her daughter; covertly he is talking about his gift to her. He indirectly tells her to thank herself, not him, for the changes that have happened. The word 'anonymous' actually tells her to forget about him. Unconsciously, she will always remember who helped her make this change, but consciously she might forget about it — and the more she forgets Brooks, the more she will hold herself responsible for her positive response to spiders. Let's look at the sentence "Something very special. Look into those eyes now, and give that gift to your child." Again, this is a reference to the beginning of the session, to the induction phase when the client was *looking* at her *special* rings that were also a *gift*. This is yet another way of creating amnesia for the therapy part of the session, and to imply that it is coming to a close.

Embedded suggestions:

- I would like you[ER] now[TA] to *look into the eyes of your child.*
- *Look into those eyes* now[TA].

Direct (posthypnotic) suggestions:

- *Look into those eyes.*

Adjunctive suggestions:

- That was just something that happened - BUT that child is never gonna have to learn what you've been through in the past.
- *Look into those eyes* now - AND *give that gift to your child.*

Embedded statements:

- Because[DM] what you've just done for yourself, now[TA] you've also done for that child.
- Now[DM] your mom couldn't help it back then.
- And[DM] that is the gift that you can give your child.
- And know[FV] that child will never know about it.
- I was thinking[TF] that the best gifts are the ones, that you don't actually get appreciation for, the ones you give anonymously almost[LS].
- You don't do it out of selfishness, or wanting kind of, you know[DM] some kind of thanks.
- It's lovely[QA] to be able[MO] to do that for your own child.
- Of course[SA], you give many gifts to your child, right[TQ]?
- Just[DA] being you, just[DA] being her mother.

Direct statements:

- Those eyes are telling you something.
- You couldn't help learning it.
- That is something so special.
- That's such a gift.

Vague language:

- Nominalisation: future, gift
- Vague adjective: beautiful, special, lovely
- Loaded word: gift
- Unspecified place: back here
- Unspecified object: something
- Comparative deletion: best
- Lost performant: don't they always tell you something those eyes

- Universal quantifier: always, never
- No personal pronoun (infinitive): it's lovely *to be able* to do that
- Permissive: you can

Presuppositions:

- Negative question:
  <u>don't they</u> always tell you something? $\supseteq$ I think they always tell you something

- Qualifying adverb:
  something <u>so</u> special $\supseteq$ something special

Various techniques:

- Future pacing: "look into those eyes now and give that gift to your child"
- Normalising: "your mom couldn't help it; you couldn't help learning it"
- Complimenting: "of course, you give many gifts to your child"

Brooks: Now, I'm going to count backwards (5 sec.) from 10 to 1. WHEN I reach the number one, you can *open your eyes.* You understand that? *You come back to this room.* WITH EACH number, *you slowly come back to this room*, just one number at a time. 10..9..8..7..6.. *slowly coming back*..5..4..3.. *starting to think about opening your eyes*..2..1 (she opens her eyes).

> Brooks brings her back from the trance by counting backwards from 10 to 1. This seems a straightforward, standard technique for bringing the client back from trance. Remember, however, how the client's fear was scaled between 1 and 10 at the beginning of the session. Counting backwards from 10 to 1 tells her unconscious mind not just to come back but also to let go of any residual fear. Throughout the session, Brooks has, in various ways, given her the message that her problem would be solved. Counting back from 10 to 1 is a final symbolic way to do that.
>
> Embedded suggestions:
>
> - <u>You can</u>[MO] *come back to this room.*

- 10..9..8..7..6 *slowly coming back.*
- 5..4..3 *starting to think about opening your eyes.*

Direct suggestions:

- *You come back to this room.*

Dependent suggestions:

- WHEN I reach the number one - you can *open your eyes.*
- WITH EACH number - *you slowly come back to this room.*

Vague language:

- Vague adverb: slowly
- No personal pronoun (gerund): slowly *coming* back; *starting* to think about opening your eyes
- Permissive: you can

Presuppositions:

- Change-of-place verb:
  You can <u>come back</u> to this room ⊇ you are not in this room now

- Repetitive cue word:
  You can come <u>back</u> to this room ⊇ you were in this room before

- Qualifying adverb:
  <u>slowly</u> come back ⊇ come back
  <u>just</u> one number at a time ⊇ one number at a time

Brooks: Wowww. (she moves her head, smiles, looks at him) Hi there.

> Normally, people say hi when they just meet someone. Saying it when a client comes out of trance implies that he or she has been away and ratifies the trance. It is also another way of referring to the beginning of the encounter and thereby enhancing amnesia.

Client: (laughs) I feel heavy.

Brooks: Hmm, that's something *that will only stay with you for a minute ... or so.* (10 sec.)

Brooks normalises her experience of heaviness. He also gives her permission to keep the heaviness (a trance phenomenon) a little longer.

Client: (leans her head back, then forward again, looks at him, smiles)

Brooks: You have beautiful eyes.

Client: Thanks. I've heard someone else say that as well.

Brooks: In fact, they look prettier with them open than with them closed.

Client: (laughs shyly).

Brooks: I will always remember them.

Again Brooks compliments her. Talking about beautiful eyes is also a way of reinforcing the posthypnotic suggestion with the beautiful eyes of her child as a trigger. The statement "I will always remember them" carries the influence of the session in to her entire future.

Embedded statements:

- In <u>fact</u>[SA] they look prettier with them open.

Direct statements:

- That's something *that will only stay with you for a minute or so.*
- You have beautiful eyes.
- I will always remember them.

Vague language:

- Unspecified time: a minute or so
- Unspecified object/event: something
- Universal quantifier: always

Client: Really weird.

Brooks: Just *take your time, take your time to come back*, okay? *Take your time to come back* (briefly turns to the audience, starts speaking with a louder voice) Okay. ... Well, you know, *the next thing for you is to spend some time wandering around the corridors here.*

The fact that she describes her experience as weird confirms her trance state.

Embedded suggestions:

- Just[DA] *take your time, take your time to come back.*
- Well[DM] you know[DM] *the next thing for you is to spend some time wandering around the corridors here.*

Direct suggestions:

- *Take your time to come back.*

Vague language:

- Vague verb: to come back
- Unspecified place: around the corridors

Presuppositions:

- Pseudo-cleft sentence:
  the next thing for you is ⊇ there is something for you

- Ordinal numeral:
  the next thing for you is ⊇ you have already done things

Client: (laughs) Yeah.

Brooks: But BEFORE you do that, uhh ... I want you to just ... in your mind, when you *think of the spider, or anything like that, anything that used to make you scared* (pointing behind her). Just *think of something now* (pointing in front of her), just to get in your mind. And tell me on a scale of, you know, 1 to 10 (indicating the scale with his left hand), remember you said it was 11 before. Tell me where, where your fear is now, AS *you think of the spider.*

Client: Nothing.

Brooks: One or zero?

Client: Zero (shaking her head as if she cannot believe it yet)

> Brooks now tests the effect of the session using scaling. Reminding her of her fear level at the start of the session ratifies the influence of the session and the effect it has created. He challenges her by asking if her fear has gone down to one or zero. Realising and saying it is really zero is another way to ratify the effect of the session.

Embedded suggestions:

- I want you to[ER] *just...think of the spider or anything like that.*
- Just[DA] *think of something now* just[DA] to get in your mind.

Dependent suggestions:

- BEFORE *you do that* - I want you to just, in your mind…
- Tell me where your fear is now - AS *you think of the spider.*

Implications:

- used to make you scared ⊃ doesn't make you scared anymore
- you said it was 11 before ⊃ it's not 11 anymore
- where your fear is now ⊃ your fear is not where it was before

Brooks: Zero. Well how did you do that?

Client: (softly speaking, smiling, and shrugging her shoulders) I don't know.

The question "How did you do that?" is not directed to her conscious mind. It is an indirect way of saying "You did it yourself"; another compliment. Her conscious mind answers, "I don't know".

Brooks: Because you're the one who did it, you worked very hard, AND let me tell you, you did a very good job.

The compliment is now given explicitly.

Client: (looks up into space).

Brooks: You look a bit puzzled.

Client: (smiling) Yeah. I don't know. It just seems really weird. I mean, it just felt as if I was...It wasn't as if I was asleep, but it was just as if... Normally I would get very nervous, but I wasn't nervous at all.

Again the client confirms having been in trance by comparing her experience to sleep and describing it as weird.

Adjunctive suggestions:

- You're the one who did it, you worked very hard - and let me tell you, you did a very good job.

Direct statements:

- You're the one who did it.
- You worked very hard.

Vague language:

- Vague verb: worked
- Mind reading: you look a bit puzzled

Presuppositions:

- Question:
  how did you do that? ⊇ you did that

Various techniques:

- Complimenting: "you worked very hard"; "you did a very good job"

Brooks: Well done.

Client: I'm nervous now (looking at the audience).

Brooks: In front of these people (pointing at the audience)?

Brooks utilises her returning nervousness by attributing it to the awareness of the audience.

Client: Yes, but I wasn't when I was out of it (out of it meaning in trance)

Brooks: They kind of disappeared, didn't they?

Client: Yeah.

Brooks: They weren't there.

Client: I could hear them.

Brooks: Yeah, but they didn't ... weren't important, didn't matter.

Client: (shaking her head) No (they didn't matter).

The client realises her unawareness of the audience during trance and thereby ratifies the latter. Brooks reinforces this ratification.

Embedded statements:

- They kind of disappeared <u>didn't they</u>[TQ]?
- But[DM] they didn't weren't important, didn't matter.

Direct statements:

- They weren't there.

Vague language:

- Mind reading: they kind of disappeared; they weren't there

Various techniques:

- Complimenting: well done

Brooks: Well, well done.

Another compliment.

Client: Shocking (smiling).

Describing her experience as shocking is another confirmation of the trance.

Brooks: Okay, I think you get yourself a cup of tea or something like that.

Client: Yeah.

Brooks: Okay. And maybe you want to spend ten minutes or fifteen minutes, for example, with Mary maybe, having a look around at the hospital corridor, AND see if you can *find some friends.*

Brooks now reorients her to the activities, other people and the external world.

Client: (Smiling) I have just seen a little flying thing just now, it went on my shoulder.

Brooks: See!

Client: Where did it go?

Brooks: I'll tell you what, friends are going to come to you, you know. Can I take my microphone back?

Client: Yeah. (taking the microphone off).

Embedded statements:

- I'll tell you what[A] friends are going to come to you, you know[DM].

Adjunctive suggestions:

- Having a look around at the hospital corridor - AND see if you can *find some friends*.

Vague language:

- Unspecified person: some friends

Immediately after the session, the client was asked to explore the corridors of the hospital to find spiders and test her response. This she did with enthusiasm, successfully making lots of new 'spider friends', even allowing them to crawl onto her hands without any recurrence of her previous fear.

Index

D

E

F

G

H

I

J

K

L

M

N

O

P

Q

R

S

T

U

V

W

Y

References

Bandler, R. (1985). *Using your brain - or a change.* Real People Press.

Bandler, R., & Grinder, J. (1975). *Patterns of Hypnotic Techniques of Milton H. Erickson Vol I.* Meta Publications.

Bandler, R., & Grinder, J. (1975). *The Structure of Magic Volume I: A Book About Language and Therapy.* Science & Behavior Books.

Bandler, R., & Grinder, J. (1981). *Trance-formations: Neuro-Linguistic Programming and the structure of hypnosis.* Real People Press.

Bannink, F. (2010). *1001 Solution Focused Questions.* New York: Norton.

De Shazer, S., & Dolan, Y. (2007). *More then Miracles: The State of the Art of Solution Focussed Brief Therapy.* Routledge.

Dilts, R. B. (1990). *Changing Beliefs Systems with NLP.* Meta Publications.

Dilts, R. B. (1999). *Sleight of mouth; The magic of conversational belief change.* Meta publications.

Dilts, R. B., Hallbom, T., & Smith, S. (1990). *Beliefs: Pathway to Health & Well-Being.* Metamorphous Press.

Ekman, P. (2003). *Emotions revealed: Understanding faces and feelings.* Orion Publishing Co.

Erickson, M. H., & Rossi, E. L. (1979). *Hypnotherapy: An exploratory casebook.* Irvington.

Erickson, M. H., & Rossi, E. L. (1980). *Indirect Forms of Suggestion. In The collected papers of Milton H. Erickson, Volume I.* Irvington.

Erickson, M. H., & Rossi, E. L. (1980a). *The nature of hypnosis and suggestions: In the collected papers of Milton H. Erickson, Volume I.* Irvington.

Erickson, M. H., & Rossi, E. L. (1980b). *Innovative Hypnotherapy. In the collected papers of Milton H. Erickson Volume IV*. Irvington.

Erickson, M. H., & Rossi, E. L. (1980c). *Two-level Communication and the Microdynamics of Trance and Suggestion: In The collected papers of Milton H. Erickson, Volume I.* Irvington.

Erickson, M. H., & Rossi, E. L. (1981). *Experiencing Hypnosis.* Irvington.

Erickson, M. H., Rossi, E. L., & Rossi, S. I. (1976). *Hypnotic Realities.* Irvington.

Farrelly, F., & Brandsma, J. F. (1981). *Provocative Therapy.* Meta Publications.

Gilligan, S. (1987). *Therapeutic Trances - The cooperation principle in Ericksonian Hypnotherapy.* Routledge.

Gordon, D. (1978). *Therapeutic Metaphors.* Meta Publications.

Haley, J. (1973). *Uncommon Therapy; The psychiatric techniques of Milton H. Erickson, M.D.* Norton.

Hall, L. M., & Bodenhamer, B. G. (1997). *Figuring out people: Reading People Using Meta-Programs.* Wales: Crown House publishing.

Hall, L. M., & Bodenhamer, B. G. (1997). *Mind-Lines: Lines for Changing Minds.* E.T. Publications.

Hill, R., & Rossi, E. L. (2017). *The Practitioner's Guide to Mirroring Hands.* Crown House Publishing.

Ledoux, J. (1996). *The emotional brain; The mysterious underpinnings of emotional life.* Simon & Schuster.

Nerin, W. F. (1986). *Family Reconstruction: Long Day's Journey into Light.* New York: Norton.

O'Connor, J. (2001). *NLP Workbook: practical guide to achieving the results you want.* HarperCollins Publisher.

O'Hanlon, W. (1987). *Taproots: Underlying Principles of Milton Erickson's Therapy and Hypnosis.* Norton.

O'hanlon, W., & Weiner-Davis, M. (1989). *In search for solutions: A new Direction in Psychotherapy.* New York: Norton.

Rossi, E. L., & Cheek, D. (1988). *Mind-Body Therapy: Methods of ideodynamic Healing in Hypnosis.* Norton.

Schiffrin, D. (1987). *Discourse markers: Studies in Interactional Sociolinguistics.* Cambridge University Press.

Shapiro, F. (2001). *Eye Movement Desensitization and Reprocessing (EMDR): Basic Principles, Protocols, and Procedures, 2nd Edition.* The Guilford Press.

Van der Kolk, B., McFarlane, A., & Weisaeth, L. (2007). *Traumatic Stress: The Effects of Overwhelming Experience on Mind, Body, and Society.* The Guilford Press.

Zeig, J. (1980). *A Teaching Seminar with Milton Erickson.* Brunner/Mazel.

Zeig, J., & Gilligan, S. (1990). *Brief Therapy; Myths, Methods & Metaphors.* Brunner/Mazel.

Lightning Source UK Ltd.
Milton Keynes UK
UKHW030627311221
396440UK00007B/569

9 789083 074603